Milk on the Side

Extended Chest/Breastfeeding in the United States

Cassandra White
Georgia State University, USA

BLOOMSBURY ACADEMIC
NEW YORK • LONDON • OXFORD • NEW DELHI • SYDNEY

BLOOMSBURY ACADEMIC
Bloomsbury Publishing Inc, 1359 Broadway, New York, NY 10018, USA
Bloomsbury Publishing Plc, 50 Bedford Square, London, WC1B 3DP, UK
Bloomsbury Publishing Ireland, 29 Earlsfort Terrace, Dublin 2, D02 AY28, Ireland

BLOOMSBURY, BLOOMSBURY ACADEMIC and the Diana logo are trademarks of
Bloomsbury Publishing Plc

First published in the United States of America 2026

Copyright © Cassandra White, 2026

Cover design: Kathi Ha
Cover image © Magda Gabriela Dumitrescu

All rights reserved. No part of this publication may be: i) reproduced or transmitted in any form, electronic or mechanical, including photocopying, recording or by means of any information storage or retrieval system without prior permission in writing from the publishers; or ii) used or reproduced in any way for the training, development or operation of artificial intelligence (AI) technologies, including generative AI technologies. The rights holders expressly reserve this publication from the text and data mining exception as per Article 4(3) of the Digital Single Market Directive (EU) 2019/790.

Bloomsbury Publishing Inc does not have any control over, or responsibility for, any third-party websites referred to or in this book. All internet addresses given in this book were correct at the time of going to press. The author and publisher regret any inconvenience caused if addresses have changed or sites have ceased to exist, but can accept no responsibility for any such changes.

A catalog record for this book is available from the Library of Congress.

ISBN: HB: 979-8-216-27722-4
PB: 979-8-216-27721-7
ePDF: 979-8-216-27724-8
eBook: 979-8-216-27723-1

Typeset by Deanta Global Publishing Services, Chennai, India
Printed and bound in the United States of America

For product safety related questions contact productsafety@bloomsbury.com.

To find out more about our authors and books visit www.bloomsbury.com and sign up for our newsletters.

Dedication

This book is dedicated to everyone who participated in my research, including my son, Ash, without whom this research would have never happened. Your willingness to allow me to share the experiences I include here has made this book so much richer.

Contents

Acknowledgments vi
List of Abbreviations x

1 Introduction 1
2 Cultural Imaginaries, Stigma, and Taboo 15
3 "Nature" and Culture in Extended Nursing 29
4 "This Is Not Your Fight!": Input from Friends and Family 51
5 Encounters with Biomedicine: Support, Shame, Stigma, and Iatrogenic Harm 69
6 "Cease and Desist": Legal Issues and EN 99
7 Lived Experiences of EN 117
8 "The Other Side of Milk": Conclusion 149

Appendix A: In-depth Interview Questions 163
Appendix B: Participant Profiles 166
Appendix C: Court Letter for Parents Practicing EN 170
Notes 172
References 175
Index 193

Acknowledgments

This part of the book was one of the most difficult to put together because I wanted to acknowledge so many people and was concerned about who I might forget, especially because this project took so many years to complete. My son, Ash, and my mom, Judy White, were two major inspirations for this book. My mom nursed me for a year, which was a significant amount of time for that era, when many babies were formula fed. When I was struggling to establish a nursing relationship with my son, she assured me that if I was unable to make it work, it did not make me any less of a mom and that my child would know that I loved him no matter what. Thanks to both of my parents, Bill and Judy White, for always encouraging me in pursuing anthropology and in basically being supportive of everything I do.

My son was essentially a co-researcher, as chest/breastfeeding was something we learned and experienced together; my autoethnographic descriptions of my experiences necessarily include him. I appreciate that now, as a teenager, he gave me permission to include stories that are also about him as a child. He has always been incredibly brave and where I might be self-conscious, he tells me not to worry so much about what other people think. Ash, you are the best son I could have imagined.

My husband, Chris DeFrancisco, has been a great source of support in everything for over three decades. He facilitated extended nursing for me in so many ways, as I discuss in other parts of this book. Thank you for everything!

Thanks to Georgia State University (GSU) undergraduate and graduate students (Margaret Sinclair, Ghazal Khaksari, Laura Lund, Cassandra Eng, Corina Sanchez, Zachary Schroeder, Brea Cooper, Nakayla Banks, Nicole Elliot, Martha Mukasa, and Heather Thaker) who collected sources and created annotated bibliographies on extended chest/breastfeeding as my student assistants and/or shared their bibliographies for their own work on chest/breastfeeding or on maternal and child health. Serving on MA committees for Brandice Evans and Les'Shon Irby's theses, which were about support systems for chest/breastfeeding, was also helpful. Thanks to GSU alum Alicia Simpson, who also invited me to be a board member for a nonprofit she started, PeaPod

Lactation and Nutrition Support, which works with underserved communities in the Atlanta area; I learned so much from this experience.

Thanks to the students and alumni (Tami Ross, Jessica Glass, Drew Colvin, and Leslie Garrett) who participated in a panel I organized for the American Anthropological Association meetings in the fall of 2024 on medical messaging, which helped me further develop my ideas for this book.

A RISE (Research Innovation and Scholarly Excellence) grant from GSU in the fall of 2022 provided course releases so that I had time to conduct post-pandemic interviews and begin serious work on data analysis and writing. Thanks to current colleagues in our wonderfully collegial Department of Anthropology at GSU (Jennifer Patico, Faidra Papavasiliou, Nicola Sharratt, Emanuela Guano, Steven Black, Bethany Turner-Livermore, Joshua Kwoka, Louis Ruprecht, Jeffery Glover, Frank L'Engle Williams, Jennie Burnet, Nicola Sharratt, Amanda Ellwanger, Kathryn Kozaitis, and Aikaterini Grigoriadou). Thanks also to Susan McCombie, now retired from GSU, who always reminded me to focus on positive examples and best practices in biomedical contexts and not just the negatives and challenges.

Special thanks to department colleagues who helped in different ways with this work: Thanks to Bethany also for suggesting my name to Jennifer Sweeney-Tookes, who in turn put me in touch with Heidi Altman, who was getting authors together for an edited volume (*Agency and Bodily Autonomy in Systems of Care*). In preparing a chapter for this volume, I had a chance to consider the main themes to come out of my research. Thanks to Jennifer Patico, who helped make this book possible in a few ways, from her own research to her support of my work as a colleague and as a chair. She also invited me to present at a conference ("Socialism, Capitalism, and Childhood"), for which she organized the Atlanta hub. Presenting at this conference helped me to refocus my energies on this project and think through some important theoretical points. Thanks to Kathryn Kozaitis for her support of me over many years as department chair. She also facilitated a flexible work environment that made it possible for me to continue with my preferred parenting choices. She also consistently inspired me as a scholar and a parent herself. Frank L'Engle Williams introduced me to the concept of attachment parenting, which we often talked about in relation to his children and his own research on fatherhood. In addition, at GSU, thanks to Densie Davidson, who coordinated an excellent "Writing Power Hour," which I participated in periodically over several years, and Wendy Simonds, for your friendship and inspiration in research and activism.

Thanks to my academic mentors, including Maxine Margolis, Randal Johnson, Gerald Murray, Adeline Masquelier, Vicki Bricker, Judie Maxwell, and William Balée, and to my first colleagues, Claudia Chang and Deborah Durham, for your support and inspiration. As always, thanks to Marsha Coker, my first grade teacher, who has been a consistent source of positivity.

Thanks to Tamar Kapner, a friend and La Leche leader who invited me to attend a meeting when I was pregnant and shared some of her knowledge. Thanks, McCalla Orso and Yolanda Chapman, for being good friends and showing up during my labor and delivery experience.

I appreciate Katherine Dettwyler, not only for her important research on breastfeeding and weaning over the course of her life's work, but for her encouragement, via email communication, of my project in its early stages. Thanks also to Fiona Jardine and Kristin Wilson, whose work has been influential in demonstrating the multiple and complex ways that people navigate child feeding.

Special thanks to Alyssa Palazzo at Bloomsbury for reaching out to me to meet at the American Anthropological Association meetings in Tampa and for her enthusiasm and support for this project. Thanks to Anna Eggers, Arun Rajakumar, and Jehanne Schweitzer at Bloomsbury for their responsiveness in answering my many questions via email.

Thanks to anonymous editors of different versions and chapters of this book, whose comments helped to make this version stronger and to Kristin Wilson and Darcia Narvaez for their thoughtful comments for the back cover. Thanks, Magda Dumitrescu, for creating such wonderful and meaningful art for my book cover.

Thanks to the amazing mom friends who raised awesome kids and have accompanied me on different parts of this parenting journey since my son was little and through high school, including Patti Ghezzi, Blair Glass, Betsy Sinclair, Amy Hines, Janna Sayer, Allison Ketchell Campbell, Ruby Hollender, Liz Yureki, Sudha Awasthi, Katherine Prato, Dagmar Ebaugh, Namita Agravat, Jennifer Weiner, Tammy and Lori Powers, and more.

Thanks to my extended family for always being supportive, including Arleen and Les Emmons; Matt and Becky DeFrancisco; Linda and Fred Setchell, Allison Forsyth, Shannon and Bill Bransford, Sherri and Mike Magnera, Sandi Brown, John and Tabitha Herchig, Alex Forsyth, Katie Marlowe, Abby Forsyth, the Fairchilds (Michael, Susie, Marnie, and Scott); Jen Skalski; Bob and Merry Shaw, Jodie Shaw, Allison Shaw, Amy Lessler; and all my nieces and nephews.

Thanks to friends, former students, friends, and colleagues I have not yet mentioned above who have regularly talked to or asked me about the progress on this work, including Rogério Rodrigues, Dana Tottenham, Kanan Mehta, Di Ciruolo, Timothy Gitzen, Julisa Rojas, Belinda Dapreis, Christine Stauber, Jessica Fairley, Candi Clark, Amber Russell, Kyla Robinson, Susan Caolo, Alex Bodkin, Miriam Peñafort, Marcelo Vieira, Juan Ruiz, Robert Lloyd, Candace Young, Moisés Lino e Silva, Monet Moutinho, Érica Sena, Erika Robb Larkins, Jenail Marshall, Rachel Kingsley, Rachel Lewis Baker, Hannah Allen, Megan Murdock, Martha Rego, Adrienne Tremblay, Stacey Schwarzkopf, Laurel and Conard Hamilton, Iffat and Ishtiaq Ali, Robbie Finch, Rebecca Nelson, Macie Orrand, Sarah Dugal, Jennifer Griffin-Yoshizawa, Carrie Furman, Elizabeth Falconi, Mark Flanagan, Clary Herrera, Emaline Laney, Zachary Russell, Courtney Davidson, Emily Gaskin, Earvin Casciano, Rachel Hall-Clifford, Rebecca Philipsborn, Maeghan Dessecker, Erika Hewitt, JohnieSue Thurman, Jessie Griggs, Marie Huamalies-Hayes, Sean Seiler, John Godwin, Laila Panjwani, Drew Moats, Kwaneya Black, Westney Allen, Juel Ables, Astrid Indigo, Md Asaduzzaman, Ademola Adeyemi, Holly Mazella, Ayesha Khan, Valerie Masutier, Teva Edwards, Hannah Spadafora, Sydney Resler, Gabriela Alvarado, Judith Justice, Kimberly Cleveland, Christian Zsilavetz, Alexis Powers, Ruth Peters, James Staples, Onika Anglin, Chancy Gatlin, Rachel Kingsley, Joy Ciofi, Cindy Lam, Scott Walker, M.A.C. Claytor, Beatriz Miranda-Galarza, Sarah Love, Kathleen Coleman, Natasha Hill, and Susan Sutton Eccher.

I wanted to add about 1,000 more people to this list, but if I missed thanking you here, I will hopefully be able to thank you in person. Thanks to every person who participated in or assisted me in this project or supported me in some way over the many years it took me to complete it!

List of Abbreviations

AAP	American Academy of Pediatrics
ABM	Academy of Breastfeeding Medicine
AFAB	Assigned Female at Birth
AMAB	Assigned Male at Birth
CDC	Centers for Disease Control and Prevention
EBF	Exclusive Breastfeeding
EN	Extended Nursing
IBCLC	International Board Certified Lactation Consultant
LLL	La Leche League
OP	Original Poster
PM	Private Message
WHO	World Health Organization
WIC	USDA's Special Supplemental Nutrition Program for Women, Infants, and Children

1

Introduction

"And that's when you know it's time to stop!" This is a phrase that many people in the United States who practice extended chest/breastfeeding and others who nurse their children from their bodies for longer than is typically considered "normal" might hear at some point. This phrase often follows an anecdote about what the indicator that it is "time to stop" should be. During the last few years when I was nursing my son, one of my physicians would ask me during annual appointments if I had weaned yet. This was brought up primarily because I was past the age when I was supposed to begin having mammograms. She said I should wait until I had weaned because imaging results in nursing parents are difficult to interpret.[1] Each year she would tell me a story about someone she knew whose nursing child once asked for "a peanut butter and jelly sandwich with a side of mommy milk." She would end the story by saying, in a joking way, "And that's when you know it's time to stop!" Her implication was that when a child can make a sophisticated verbal request like this and when they can eat "a sandwich," they no longer "need" to be chest/breastfeeding. At first, I would laugh along and joke and say something like, "my son will probably keep nursing until he's in college."

When my son was five and my physician repeated this story, I decided to say something different in response. I said that I was thinking of conducting formal research on extended nursing and that I had learned it is not uncommon with child-led weaning,[2] in which children wean when they are ready, for children to continue to nurse past the age of five. I mentioned that there is no solid evidence-based information to link milestones like walking or talking to the need to wean. This turned into a very positive interaction, in which she seemed to really listen to what I was saying and said this was a perspective she had not considered. This interaction made me wish I had spoken up more often, nursed in public more often, and been more open and less fearful of the stigma associated with nursing a child much longer than is typical in the United States.

After more than five years of nursing my son (2007–12), without access to a large community of others who were practicing extended chest/breastfeeding at that time, I considered just writing an autoethnographic account, applying an anthropological lens to write about and analyze my own experiences. I wanted to write about why my husband and I made certain parenting decisions, to give examples of stigma I had encountered and support I received, and to discuss all the weird and unexpected aspects of nursing a child who had been asking for sandwiches for years before he stopped asking for "milk on the side." As an anthropologist, I felt that in all those years, I was engaged in participant observation, and I had been actively taking a critical perspective on my experiences. However, I was interested in seeing and understanding the experiences of others who practiced extended chest/breastfeeding, and I decided to conduct anthropological research on this topic in the United States. This work included primarily "digital ethnography" (anthropological research in online spaces) on social media platforms, engaging in online communities that have tens of thousands of people who practice extended nursing in the United States, and in other online spaces. I also conducted a small set of in-depth interviews with parents practicing extended nursing, and I kept in touch with many of them over several years. Hearing stories from other parents and caregivers allowed me to consider issues that did not come up in my own experience of nursing, including medical and legal issues that some parents face in relation to this practice and child-led weaning and pandemic-related experiences of chest/breastfeeding and childcare. My interactions with the growing community of people who nurse for longer than is typical in the United States have also helped me identify possible applications of this research to public health and to the protection of parents' and children's legal rights and personal freedoms.

Terminology

In this research, I focused on parents/caregivers who fed a child human milk from their bodies for two years or more, which I define as "extended" for the purposes of this study. I use "prolonged" sometimes in place of extended, but I more typically use "extended" in part because it is widely used on social media sites, and it reflects the popular perceptions of the act of chest/breastfeeding toddlers and older children in the United States. "Extended" in reference to nursing is a relative term that implies something that has gone beyond what is normal or typical; in retrospect, particularly after learning about the stigma people faced in nursing their children even before they had gotten close to their second birthdays, I could have chosen one year or even less for what is popularly considered "extended" in the United States, but I was thinking of World Health Organization (WHO) recommendations of "two years and beyond," which has since been adopted by the American Academy of Pediatrics (AAP) (Meek et al. 2022). I did not focus on other forms of feeding children human milk (e.g., exclusive pumping and bottle feeding of human milk); these practices may also carry a stigma, as has been discussed by Jardine (2019, 2020a) and Wilson (2018), I was interested in the stigmatized aspects of feeding a child directly from the body, though some of my participants combined bottle feeding and chest/breastfeeding.

In seeking to be gender inclusive, I refer in part to a statement by the Academy of Breastfeeding Medicine (ABM), which recommends the use of both "breastfeeding" and "chestfeeding" to describe the practice of feeding a child with human milk from one's body (Bartick et al. 2021). Many nonbinary or transmasculine people prefer "chestfeeding," or, occasionally "bodyfeeding" (Sussex 2021). It is also possible for a cisgender man or an AMAB ("assigned male at birth") transgender woman to produce milk and nurse their children (Bertollo 2024;Swaminathan 2007), although hormone supplements are usually required to produce enough milk for an infant's needs (Reisman and Goldstein 2018). Both breasts (and milk ducts) are anatomical features of all human bodies, but as Bartick et al. noted,

> most desexed or gender-inclusive terms do not have equivalent meaning to the words they replace. For example, in medical terminology, breasts refer to both the male and female body part. "Chest" is often substituted but has a different anatomical meaning and thus is not used this way in medical settings. (2021: 2)

The association of the term "breast" with femininity and cisgender women (AFAB or "assigned female at birth") is one reason why the term "chestfeeding" is preferred by some; transgender men or nonbinary people may have trauma and dysphoria associated with breasts or may have completed chest masculinization or top surgery and no longer see themselves as having "breasts."

In online groups where I conducted research, members sometimes used the abbreviation EBF to refer to extended breastfeeding, but in the academic literature on breastfeeding, EBF is typically used to refer to "exclusive breastfeeding" (meaning only human milk until solid foods are introduced). I also wanted to be inclusive of people who prefer the term "chestfeeding." I crowdsourced for some opinions in online groups about abbreviations and got suggestions such as XBF or ExtBF/CF and FTN (Full-term Nursing). "Full-term" is also relative and might be synonymous with the idea of a "natural" time for weaning, which can also be a problematic concept, as I discuss in more detail in Chapter 3. "Long-term" was another option (used by Tomori et al. 2016). In this book, I have chosen to use "extended nursing" and the abbreviation EN throughout the book.

Bartick et al. (2021) suggested "lactating persons" for people who are chest/breastfeeding, and I also use this term occasionally, along with the general phrase "people who practice EN." One of my interview participants who acknowledged the importance of gender neutral language in her own practice as a lactation consultant and pediatric nutritionist used the term "feeding person" when discussing nursing parents. Some scholars suggest the use of the word "mother" could be gender-identity neutral if used "as a verb" (Chandler 2007, cited in O'Reilly 2010: 5), implying that "mothering" practices can be done by anyone. Andrea O'Reilly, associated with creating motherhood studies as a research focus, has suggested that while patriarchal definitions of mothers and motherhood are limiting, a contemporary feminist perspective of who can be "mothers" (she uses the term "good mothers" here) can include

> noncustodial, poor, single, old, young, queer, trans, and "working" mothers; likewise, the biological category of mother itself is expanded so as to allow for other nonbiological identities of maternity such as other-mothers—grandmothers and mentors—and fathers. (2010: 8)

However, since "mother" and "mothering" are terms associated with femininity and not terms with which everyone who practices EN identifies, in this book, I use more neutral language, often using "parents" or "caregivers" when talking generally. In referring to research participants who mentioned the term they use for their relationship with their child, I use their terms; where someone identified themselves or a partner as "mother," for example, I use that term.

Methods

A colleague and friend (anthropologist Dr. Moisés Lino e Silva) wrote on a social media post that, "all ethnography is, at least partially, autoethnographic. At the same time, no ethnography can possibly be exclusively autoethnographic" (used with permission). Even with autoethnography, in which your anthropological research is focused on your own experience, you are still interpreting your experiences within the context of your background, so even if you were to write solely about your experience, you are still writing about your cultural milieu and about those with whom you interact. This project began as autoethnography. For the autoethnographic portion of this research, based on the time I spent nursing my son, I was doing informal data gathering on comments and actions of family and friends, societal norms for both chest/breastfeeding and EN, and healthcare professionals' comments and perspectives when I mentioned I was "still" nursing (especially after my son was no longer an infant). These years also included traveling to conferences, academic work, and living for brief periods abroad while directing two summer study abroad programs in Brazil. As our nursing journey neared its end, I felt compelled as an anthropologist to learn about and share the experiences of other people who have chest/breastfed for longer than what is typically perceived as "normal" in the United States.

It was only at the very end of my own nursing experience that I started to come across parenting groups on Facebook and found groups specifically dedicated to chest/breastfeeding and to EN. I became aware of what a great resource these could be for parents and of what incredible sources of ethnographic data were contained in posts and comments. Others have discussed the value of these online communities related to chest/breastfeeding challenges. In a chapter on her own struggle to get nursing established and later continue beyond what was considered "normal" in her family, writing professor Dionne Irving wrote about how the "village" she was hoping for in her own family and in-person community did not materialize. As a Black woman living in the United States, she wrote about how she had to contend with not only the typical sexualization of breasts but the hypersexualization and fetishization of Black women's bodies. She said that ultimately, it was her "electronic village" that helped her the most, including "the networks of other women of colour grappling with their bodies and with the politics attendant to feeding your child as a black mother . . . who made this community feel like a safe space, an embrace" (2018: 140). This village was comprised of online chest/breastfeeding support groups on Facebook for Black women and women of color. Fiona Jardine (2020b), in analyzing survey results from over 2,400 participants in several countries among those who chose to exclusively pump milk to feed their children, found that online support groups were key in helping people answer complicated questions that healthcare professionals were often not providing. Black et al. (2020) also noted that online support groups can assist people in meeting their nursing duration goals because they are accessible at all hours. As one of my interviewees (Sam, a white woman who was also a lactation consultant) said, in referring to online resources, "People can be in a panic [about chest/breastfeeding] and get immediate results." I wound up focusing much of my time in this research engaged in observing and participating in these online communities.

In 2012, I received Institutional Review Board (IRB) approval for a qualitative research project that turned into over a decade of digital ethnographic research on multiple internet platforms, complemented by fourteen formal, in-depth interviews (see Appendix A for interview questions). For digital ethnographic research, approaches outlined by Pink et al. (2015: 8–14) in their book (*Digital Ethnography: Principles of Practice*) align closely with mine. These include: the acknowledgment of the different ways that one can engage with the digital world; the concept of "non-digital-centricness," or moving away from the idea of "media as the focus of media research" but seeing it as the setting and context in which people are interacting (2015: 9); "openness," the idea that the internet is an "unbounded" space where we can communicate with people from anywhere in the world and where we also create relationships and communities with those with whom we connect online; the importance of self-reflection on the part of ethnographers in this constantly shifting landscape; and unorthodox approaches, with an "attention to alternative forms of communicating" (2015: 13). As an anthropologist, I find social media to be an incredible font of ethnographic data. A single post or thread can serve as a kind of focus group, often bringing in perspectives and experiences of hundreds of people in a short period of time. There are single TikTok videos that succinctly encapsulate the experiences and stigma associated with EN in a format that is arguably more accessible and effective in communicating messages than any academic text. Though social media can be siloed and affected by algorithms that determine who sees what and who is exposed to the messages that are presented, research in online spaces allowed me to observe and read a much wider range of experiences of EN than would have been possible with traditional ethnography.

Between 2012 and 2024, I also interacted through private messaging (PM) with several dozen individuals; these interactions included conversations about a post or comment and my requests to paraphrase something they posted (for these, I would request consent and send them a copy of an IRB approved form). I assigned pseudonyms to those participants whose stories I have included in this book (see also Appendix B). One of the limitations to my approach of observing and requesting permission to paraphrase comments in online spaces was that I did not collect extensive information on participants' demographic information, other than racial identity and region of residence in the United States.³ When discussing posts made by people who have a public page (not a personal page, but, for example, a public Facebook page or blog, or whose public social media page has also been featured by news outlets), I do discuss additional identifiable information in the book. There were a few cases in which an interaction that was initiated through online support groups resulted in me conducting a formal in-depth interview. For some participants who I had initially contacted about one of their posts or comments, I also wound up staying in touch via Messenger over a few years to get updates about their situations; this was most common for people who faced custody and visitation issues related to EN.

I spent extensive time in virtual data-gathering activities across several social media support groups, pages, and accounts (primarily on Facebook and Instagram, and, beginning in 2021, TikTok and Reddit) for chest/breastfeeding, EN, gentle weaning, attachment parenting, general parenting, and even some groups dedicated to cats who accompany lactating parents as they practice chest/breastfeeding. I followed and observed comments on social media sites that were run by individuals who identified as doulas, midwives, parenting bloggers/experts, and more. Many of the Facebook support groups were private in that they required approval for membership. Sites included in this research were in English and mostly had participants from the United States, though occasionally there would be participation from parents in the United Kingdom, Canada, and Australia as well as English-speaking members who lived or were living in other parts of the world. Over twelve years, I estimate that I have spent close to 2,000 hours as a participant observer online, reading through several thousand posts. I also regularly posted comments in online support groups. For data management, I took notes and kept a file with excerpts of posts and comments, eventually organizing them by topics and themes that emerged (e.g., "experiences with pediatricians" or "stigmatizing attitudes from family members"), which led to the organization of the chapters and subsections in this book.

For this project, I also conducted fourteen in-depth interviews with parents who practiced EN. I conducted five in-person, audio-recorded interviews in 2017 (at coffee shops, private homes, and in a campus office) and nine in-depth interviews between 2022 and 2024 via WebEx or Zoom, which provided an interesting perspective on EN and how the Covid-19 pandemic affected the experience of nursing and caregiving of young children. I recruited interviewees among people through my own social network and through online parenting and EN groups. In my in-depth interview sample, all were eighteen and older, born and raised in the United States and living in different US states, primarily in the Southeast and Midwest, at the time of our interviews. I asked people to self-identify in terms of race and ethnic identity; nine participants self-identified as "white," "Caucasian," or "of European descent"; one as Asian American (with parents born in India); one as "Black and Mexican/Mexican American" (mother is from Mexico, father is Black/African American); one as "Black/African American," and one as "multiracial" (mother is white, father is Black). The majority were middle class to upper middle class at the time of interview, though a few grew up in lower middle class families. All of them used she/her pronouns, though when I began the research in 2012, I did not ask about cisgender versus transgender identity or their sexuality. One participant volunteered the fact that she does not "identify her sexuality" but "was married to a cis het man" at the time of interview. Interviewees ranged in age from 28 to 47 at the time of the interviews. Every participant in in-depth interviews had completed a college degree and most had graduate degrees and certificates. Appendix B has brief profiles of each in-depth interview participant along with assigned pseudonyms; I also use pseudonyms for some of the participants with whom I exchanged PMs (but with whom I did not do full in-depth interviews). When I introduce participants in this book, I try to include some of their demographic information when I first mention them or in cases where aspects of their identity are relevant to the context.

A criterion for interviewees was that they had nursed at least one child for two years or more, but participants had a range of experiences with infant and child feeding and weaning. Carter (1995) and Copelton et al. (2010) have mentioned that the perceived dichotomy between nursing versus formula-feeding is artificial. Some parents nurse for a short period of time before switching to formula or use formula to supplement their own supply, and some may nurse one child exclusively but practice formula-feeding with another. Among my interview participants, a few had weaned one or more of their children before two years and/or used formula at some point. For example, Paige, who identified as white and grew up in the rural Southeast, was in high school when she got pregnant with her first child and said that at the time, her supply was low and "no one gave me any kind of, you know, breastfeeding consultation or people to reach out to receive breastfeeding services." She tried pumping but "wasn't producing enough." However, with her second child, she had more support and resources and was able to nurse for two years.

This project was not a longitudinal study by design, but the research period was prolonged in part because of various responsibilities I had as a parent and that I took on in service and teaching roles, research, and writing unrelated to this project, though of course time management and the pandemic played parts in this as well. In the fall of 2022, I received a grant from my university that allowed me the time to pull together the results of many years of online research, to conduct additional in-depth interviews, and to complete a more systematic analysis of topics and themes that came up on social media sites. The silver lining of the length of time over which I completed this work meant that I had a chance to capture some of the changes that have taken place in the United States (and globally) over this time, including the Covid-19 pandemic and shifts in social media.

A Note on Anonymity and Confidentiality in Online Research

Research in online settings is no longer new territory for ethnographers. There are some protocols for doing this type of ethnographic research, but standard methods can be difficult to lay out since the internet and social media platforms change rapidly. Each platform is very different in terms of how comments and stories are presented and how privacy and anonymity are or are not maintained. The majority of my time was spent on private Facebook support groups that require members to answer membership questions and follow established rules. In private groups, the expectation is that participants' posts and comments not be quoted or shared outside of the site, so much of the data gathering I did in these groups was about identifying common themes. Public groups are viewable by anyone; these public comments might be fair game for research use, but participants do not necessarily comment with the idea that their words will be quoted verbatim in academic publications. Within Facebook groups, there are search features that make it easy to search for topics and terms and to find specific posts and comments, including my own over several years. This both facilitated my research and made me aware that citing anything someone says online without paraphrasing means that anyone can easily search and find people's individual comments. As I learned more about some of the legal issues that people who practice EN can face in custody hearings in particular, I tried to be cautious about how I was presenting the stories people shared online or with me directly. Direct quotations from social media sources are only used in this book if they are from a published article or public-facing page or blog. I have paraphrased comments and posts for which I have obtained consent to include in the research so that they are not searchable.

In some cases, dozens of posts or comments expressed the same sentiment, and occasionally for this book, I have distilled multiple comments that express the same idea into a representative statement, which both has the effect of generalizing an experience and making it more difficult to trace experiences back to an individual. This tends to erase how individuals' identities might play a part in EN experiences, but these representative statements do reflect EN online support group members of different backgrounds and from different parts of the United States.

Positionality

A reviewer of a grant proposal for this research suggested that it would be impossible for me to carry out research on this topic from an unbiased perspective because I practiced EN myself. My experience of nursing my child for longer than is typical in the United States certainly did affect how I view and understand this practice, though I have tried to be conscious of ways in which this experience and other aspects of my identity (often referred to as "positionality" in the social sciences) could affect my analysis of the data. No research can be completely unbiased or objective; we all bring our experiences and aspects of our identity to our data gathering, but this does not render the research invalid. Our positionality impacts the questions we ask and our interpretation of the data, and my "insider" perspective on this topic shaped the research questions and the themes on which this book is based, but I tried to remain open to the idea that other people might have very different perspectives and experiences.

I was aware of the set of privileges that shaped my experience and facilitated both initiation of breastfeeding and being able to feed my son almost on-demand for several years. I am a white/of mostly European descent, cisgender, heterosexual woman, and I am middle class in terms of income, with moderate generational wealth that facilitated home ownership by the time my child was two. I have had stable employment and decent health insurance as a college professor since I received my PhD. My partner (husband), who also has a PhD in anthropology and works as a part-time university instructor, was mostly a stay-at-home dad during the years when our son was young. Despite the fact that my institution did not offer any paid parental leave, our son was born at the end of the academic year, so I was able to stay home for the summer months after giving birth. Once I returned to work in the fall, my husband was able to bring our son to campus between my classes during the first year of his life so that I could nurse. I was privileged in having my own office for privacy and a collegial department in which there was no resistance to having children on campus. I also had colleagues who studied parenting practices and several who were parents of young children themselves.

When I was nursing, I missed out on being a part of online communities of people who have similar experiences; some of them existed at the time, but I did not think to look for them until after my son was weaned. These groups would have helped immensely in validating that we were not the only ones practicing EN. I did have some friends and family members who nursed for more than two years, but at five years, I felt that I was in unknown territory. Still, another privilege that greatly impacted my experience was the anthropological knowledge that EN was practiced in other cultures across time and space, and I had the skills to investigate this on my own through accessing the academic literature.

Limitations

I attempted to capture diverse perspectives and experiences of EN through both interviews and digital ethnographic research, but my study is not necessarily representative of everyone practicing EN in the United States. I had a relatively small number of in-depth interview participants, and though there is some level of diversity in terms of racial and ethnic identity among my interviewees, the majority of participants identified as white and middle class with an undergraduate degree or higher. In online groups, I had a chance to observe perspectives represented across a wider range of identities, though in seeking general themes in support groups, I was not always able to collect extensive information on how some of the differences in individual identity played a part in the EN experience. Some parenting and chest/breastfeeding groups I followed that were targeted to specific minoritized identities were helpful in providing different perspectives, but they were not focused on EN specifically. Support groups and other forums where people post online also do not represent everyone who practices EN. Still, through this research, I was able to explore experiences that were beyond the limited scope of my own autoethnographic experience.

Organization of the Book

In the next chapter, I discuss the concept of cultural imaginaries related to childhood and parenting and how they are bolstered by popular beliefs, stigma, and taboos associated with EN in the United States. I include a brief, intersectional history that highlights the roles that social class, racial identity, the legacy of slavery, capitalism (including the industrial production and distribution of formula and baby food), second wave feminism, and neoliberalism played in the development of EN stigma. In Chapter 3, I discuss the variety of practices cross-culturally related to child nutrition and weaning (in both humans and our nonhuman primate relatives), and I address the problematic aspects of constructing EN as a wholly "natural" practice or as "unnatural"/ "abnormal". Chapters 4–6 deal with popular beliefs about EN that manifest in different settings and in different types of relationships; the stories and narratives included in these chapters include examples of both supportive attitudes and actions as well as displays of not only disdain and disgust but often horror and moral panic about the implications for children's psychological, emotional, and physical health and development. In Chapter 4, I focus on how beliefs about the appropriate age to wean are constructed and communicated by friends and family members, who often express unsolicited opinions in person and virtually. In Chapter 5, I give examples of stigma related to EN in healthcare settings and the iatrogenic (originating from or generated by the medical encounter) harm that can come from this stigma. Chapter 6 is about the legal implications of EN and how knowledge gaps about EN within the US court system can strip parents who practice EN of their agency (or the ability to make decisions and act on them), including in divorce and custody settlements, jail or prison sentences, and jury duty service. The consequences of the behaviors and speech of family, healthcare providers, and legal authorities on people who practice EN and their children will be discussed in these chapters as well.

I switch gears a bit in Chapter 7 to focus on the lived experience of EN beyond the frustrations that come about from other people's unsolicited advice or mandates to wean. This chapter focuses on some of the positive perceptions and experiences among people who practice EN, the physical and emotional challenges that people who nurse their children for several years face, coping strategies that allow people to manage stigma and retain their agency (and their children's agency) in a society that makes fully child-led weaning almost impossible, and the aspects of the EN experience that are humorous within the community of EN parents and caregivers. I conclude the book with some reflections about the future of EN in the United States, including how the Covid-19 pandemic has affected parenting and has in some ways opened new doors for people who may want to practice child-led weaning, while creating new parenting struggles as well, and how recent political changes are affecting families and choices about EN.

2

Cultural Imaginaries, Stigma, and Taboo

Practices that are stigmatized and constructed as taboo lend themselves to myth and mystery, in part because they are hidden from much of society. Every day on EN support groups on social media, there are multiple posts that illustrate stigmatizing attitudes and beliefs about EN that are heard from healthcare providers, partners, in-laws, colleagues, friends, and strangers. I paid close attention to posts and videos where people vented about what they (EN parents) saw as not just inaccurate but "nonsensical." Once in a while, parents or bloggers would create a post asking people about different beliefs they have heard; for example, they might post: "Wild comments you've heard about extended nursing. Go!," often starting with an example from their own experience, and this would be followed by dozens of examples of things commenters have heard from others about why EN is harmful or a waste of time. These beliefs about chest/breastfeeding and weaning are typically presented as common sense or as science-based information that suggests what is "natural" or "normal," but many of these popular cognitive models of EN emerged within a wider cultural and historical framework that has resulted in EN seeming "out of place." A number of historical events, to be explored in this chapter, contributed to the rise of a "cultural imaginary" in the United States in which prolonged childcare is seen to limit individual productivity in a capitalist economy.

Benedict Anderson was one of the first to write about widely accepted "imaginaries" (in his book, *Imagined Communities*) (2006) to discuss the development of nation-states and the artificial lines and myth-building of concepts that led to the creation of national borders and nationalist frameworks. Others have used terms like "social" or "cultural imaginaries" to talk about other types of generally shared beliefs that play into a particular agenda. Philosopher Charles Taylor used the term "social imaginaries" to describe the

> ways people imagine their social existence, how they fit together with others, how things go on between them and their fellows, the expectations that are

normally met, and the deeper normative notions and images that underlie these expectations. (2003: 23)

He wrote that he used the term "imaginary" because when "ordinary people 'imagine' their social surroundings . . . this is often not expressed in theoretical terms, but is carried in images, stories, and legends" (2003: 23). For Taylor, a social imaginary is "shared by large groups of people, if not the whole society" (2003: 23). In their discussion of imaginaries of climate change, Levy and Spicer wrote that imaginaries are related not only to "the ways in which institutions and economic activity are organized and structured," but also to how "people think they *ought* to be organized and structured" (2013: 660).

Popular or folk beliefs (the "stories and legends" that Taylor mentioned) about EN, feeding practices, and weaning could also be understood as "explanatory models" that, I argue, uphold a broader social or cultural imaginary about childhood and independence in the United States. Medical anthropologist and psychiatrist Arthur Kleinman was the first to use the term "explanatory models" to describe how people explained or understood health, illness, and the body (Kleinman 1978). These cognitive models might be informed by what people learn from those around them as they grow up, from their interpretation of science, what they see online, and much more. Most of the explanatory models discussed in this book purport developmental, psychological, physical, or moral harm or illness that could arise from weaning "too late." In many cases, these models are expressed as having a scientific basis, as people link them to biological or psychological "facts," or they are voiced by people (e.g., healthcare professionals) whose supposed authoritative knowledge is assumed to be truth. As will be discussed in Chapter 3, attempts to apply the scientific model to determining appropriate or "natural" parenting practices or weaning times for humans can also be problematic. However, the assertions that are wielded in the service of coercion of parents and children to wean before they are ready or to change their EN-related parenting practices have a great deal of weight in the contemporary United States.

I suggest that the overarching cultural imaginary that beliefs/explanatory models about the appropriate duration of chest/breastfeeding is informed by neoliberal[1] capitalist imperatives or demands. One of the goals of a neoliberal society is for children to become independent and productive citizens and for their parents to maintain productivity and "value" to a capitalist society through their work/labor. Thorley (2021) has argued that within a neoliberal economy, chest/breastfeeding in general is not valued because it is not associated with a monetary value and involves invisible labor. Within a neoliberal society, independence is linked to weaning, and in the popular imagination, children who exhibit other signs of maturity (such as other developmental milestones) but are still nursing are thought to suffer long-term negative consequences. The explanatory models about EN that serve to compel people to wean before they or their children are ready could be understood as part of the hegemony, or overarching societal influence, of capitalism and particularly the neoliberal agenda.

In an article on neoliberalism and childhood, Peter Moss and Guy Roberts-Holmes suggest that the neoliberal agenda is one that seeks to ensure that "children achieve predefined outcomes" (2022: 97) and that there is time pressure in childrearing and childhood education in a neoliberal system. This idea of time pressure was also evident in my interviewees' comments about pressures they heard from others about the need to wean "right away" or "cold turkey." In another publication, I have noted that one of my research participants, who was compelled by both her mother and doctors to wean before she and her son were ready, talked about the feeling of a "clock looming over" her and her son (White 2024: 85). The desired outcome for children in a neoliberal world, according to Moss and Roberts-Holmes, is to become "an economic being—*homo economicus*, self-interested and competitive, independent and self-reliant" (2022: 97). EN is perceived to delay the development not only of the child as the "ideal neoliberal subject," but of the chest/breastfeeding parent whose economic productivity is potentially decreased. Lindsey Reuben, in an article titled, "Breastfeeding Against the Clock: Motherhood on the Tenure Track," describes the "neoliberal workplace" as one that "condenses the heterogeneity of time into a linear clock that orders the forward movement of beings and things in the world in the name of capital" (2022: Online) and does not account for the complexities of care that are needed with nursing, either short or long term.

The voicing of anxieties about EN (by people who have not engaged in this practice) serves to uphold contemporary norms and to critique alternative ways of parenting. Although I did not quantify the frequency of different beliefs related to EN, I identified the following assertions that were commonly discussed by participants in interviews and people in online spaces:

Developmental/Milestone-Related

"Natural" milestones for weaning are when children:

- Get their first teeth ("when they can bite").
- Can talk/first words/being able to talk (specifically "when they can ask for it").
- Develop certain motor skills (being able to tug and pull at a breast or shirt or "unbutton a blouse"; if they can "drink from a cup").
- Start solid foods.
- Can walk.

Psychological/Social Consequences of EN

Children should not nurse for too long because:

- They will become experts at manipulation.
- EN is overindulgent parenting that will "spoil" the child.
- The child will never gain independence or learn to self-soothe.
- The nursing parent gets sexual or emotional gratification from chest/breastfeeding.

Other Explanatory Models

- As a child gets older, chest/breastfeeding is "just for comfort."
- Breast milk loses all nutritional and caloric value and becomes "like water" after a certain amount of time (often "after 6 months").
- EN causes physical health problems.

Most of the negative comments that people who practice EN hear often are variations on the above beliefs.

One parent-created meme on an online support group for EN illustrated some of these popular beliefs and how they fit into a wider cultural imaginary about the need to wean when children show other signs of maturity. In the meme, the caption suggested that others had said to her (the parent) that if her kids could eat a vegetable (which they did), they did not need breast milk. She posted a photo of her children tandem nursing (nursing more than one child) with an image of a raw vegetable with eyes pasted over her head. The belief/explanatory model to which she was responding in a creative and humorous way (to a receptive audience of other EN parents who understood the context) is the idea that if children can eat solid foods, they no longer need human milk. The introduction of solid foods and the motor skills required to eat a vegetable with a fork could be seen as developmental milestones that symbolize (for others) a need to wean. In the United States, perhaps more than in other cultural contexts, there is almost a shared assumption that children do not like vegetables. In anthropologist Jennifer Patico's research on middle class parenting and anxiety related to food choices and parenting decisions, she noted that "vegetables were the category of food most universally understood [by parents] as desirable and, perhaps, as most difficult to get children to eat enough of" (2020: 43), which is a belief that seems to be common in the United States. One of Patico's interlocutors,[2] for example, said that her five-year-old child prefers choices like okra that she had brought in for a class snack, but the okra was rejected by the other kids; she said that her kids "do not 'do kid foods,'" implying that vegetables and non-junk food choices are more "adult" choices (Patico 2021: 118). In the example from the Facebook post, people who voiced this sentiment about when to wean could be expressing a discomfort with children who were exhibiting maturity and sophistication through eating a vegetable (illustrated as a raw vegetable, not mushed baby food) but also continuing to nurse from their mother's body. Throughout this book, I will return to the concept of these popular beliefs/explanatory models about weaning and the wider imaginary they support as they relate to the variety of contexts in which stigma is felt by and enacted against people who practice EN.

Stigma and EN

Much of this book is dedicated to describing the experience of stigma associated with EN and understanding how it is perpetuated. Stigma is a complicated topic and has been a thread that connects much of my research since the 1990s, including ethnographic research on Hansen's disease/leprosy in Brazil and the United States; racial identity among Brazilians in the United States; health and immigration; and personal experiences of paranormal or nonempirical phenomena. At an international workshop on stigma held in Soesterberg, the Netherlands in 2002, with people who worked with multiple health-related conditions, I had a chance to think through the complexities of stigma, a term and concept that sociologist Erving Goffman described as an "attribute that is deeply discrediting" (1963: 3). While Goffman made several valuable contributions to discussions of stigma, others have looked to explore further nuances of how stigma operates. Goffman did acknowledge that "deeply discrediting" could be understood within a particular social and cultural context. However, even within a particular culture, there are a number of factors that determine not only if but how stigma can impact someone's life.

Richard Parker and Peter Aggleton (2003) discussed the how HIV/AIDS stigma is connected to structural inequalities that both contribute to and reinforce attitudes about people with HIV/AIDS who are already marginalized because of other aspects of their identity. James Staples (2011), an anthropologist who has focused his research on Hansen's disease/leprosy in India, also called for an approach to understanding stigma that considers individual life circumstances, including not only factors related to race, class, and gender, but also how the associated roles play out in the context of people's daily lives. Staples pointed out that stigma needs to be understood as a more "dynamic" process as opposed to a condition that is inherently stigmatizing:

> [W]e need to understand the everyday life worlds within which people stigmatise and are stigmatised, because, contrary to how stigma might be presented as a constant, it is not something uniformly applied to leprosy affected people across different contexts. At different stages of the life cycle and within different networks of relationships discrimination takes different forms. (2011: 92)

With EN in the United States, there are complex and intersecting structural and individual factors that affect the experience of stigma and (especially) the consequences of this stigma, which could range from weaning before the parent and child are ready to losing custody of or access to one's child. Racial identity, gender identity, social class, and access to different forms of capital, as described by Pierre Bourdieu (1986), all play large parts in how stigma associated with EN winds up being felt or enacted. The "social capital" or networks (e.g., through in-person nursing groups, like La Leche League [LLL], or groups and other resources found on social media platforms) to which people have access also have an impact on "cultural capital," or knowledge that might help them navigate different family, medical, and legal systems that might in turn affect their decisions or ability to continue EN despite external pressures to wean. I have been able to draw on the symbolic capital of a doctorate, a university affiliation, and formal research experience to advocate for myself when I was practicing EN and later in attempts to assist others as an "expert" on EN for legal cases. Access to "economic capital" (monetary wealth) in the short term and through generational sources also has an impact on EN (e.g., in the ability to make choices about childcare and work).

The stigma that exists surrounding EN is not universal (as will be discussed in more detail in Chapter 3, which includes a discussion of practices related to weaning and EN cross-culturally). Anthropologist Mary Douglas' writings on stigma and taboo offered a way to understand some of the symbolic reasons that certain behaviors or attributes are stigmatized. Other social scientists who have looked at EN (Andrews 2022, in Norway; Dowling and Pontin 2017, in the United Kingdom) have also found Douglas' work useful in understanding the experiences of those who practice it. In *Purity and Danger* (1966), Douglas described how things that fall outside of existing categories of what is considered normative, standard, or default tend to be stigmatized. For example, and of relevance to a discussion of EN, if the "default" for personhood is a cisgender man, as in many patriarchal societies, subsequently many aspects of humanity that are understood to fall outside of that category are more likely to be subject to taboo and stigma. In patriarchal societies, then, menstrual fluid, pregnancy, breast milk, and many other bodily states and substances associated with women are constructed as symbolically polluted and contaminating to others. Substances and practices associated with women and femininity are subject to taboo in many patriarchal societies (including smaller scale societies), though these taboos do not extend to public chest/breastfeeding in all societies.

In the United States (and globally), there are historical factors that have led to the extreme aversion that many people have when seeing or hearing about a nursing child who can stand on their own, ask for milk, and in other ways resemble a grown "person." Before the development of baby formula and bottles, if mothers had difficulties nursing, they might turn to other family members or to a wet nurse. Cross-culturally, there have also been alternatives used to human milk that were sometimes given to infants, including animal milk and supplementation with solids in early infancy. In the United States, social class and racial identity have also played a significant role in chest/breastfeeding tasks. Before the development of formula, upper-class white families often outsourced infant feeding to wet nurses.

During the era of chattel slavery in the United States, Black women often served as wet nurses to slaveowners' children in plantation settings, which also restricted their ability to nurse their own infants (Freeman 2020). Black parents are less likely than others in the United States to initiate chest/breastfeeding in the contemporary context, in part because of this legacy as well as a reluctance that also stems from colonial and post-colonial representations and images depicting African women with nursing children at their breasts, often unclothed (which was conflated with the idea of "primitiveness," "less evolved," and "closer to nature"). Sociologist Linda Blum, in interviews with African American working-class women in the last decade of the twentieth century, noted that they "spoke with intense feeling to reject the animality of breastfeeding and the exposure of such sexualized body parts" (1999: 193). Blum suggested that while "'nature' may be used to exalt white women, it has overwhelmingly been used to dehumanize African American mothers" (1999: 193). In a study by DeVane-Johnson et al. (2018) involving focus group research with African American women at churches, hair salons, and nursing group meetings in the United States, several participants brought up the historical issues of wet nursing during slavery and the "mammy" figure/stereotype as reasons for discomfort with chest/breastfeeding.

During the nineteenth century, the production of glass bottles and nipples made of rubber, along with Louis Pasteur's discoveries that led to better practices of sterilization and the development of artificial formula, of which there were several brands available in the West by the late 1800s, all set the stage for a major shift in the way infants and young children were fed (Stevens et al. 2009: 36; Thulier 2009). Pasteurization also allowed for the marketing of cow's milk for infants and children (Wolf 2003). The widespread distribution and marketing of infant formula in the twentieth century probably had the most significant impact on breastfeeding/chestfeeding practices and led to the drastic drop in the number of babies who ever received breast milk in the United States. In the 1930s, over 70 percent of "first-born infants [were] breastfed at birth," with 45 percent still nursing after three months, compared with only 28 percent "breastfed at birth" in 1970, and 8 percent at three months (Thulier 2009: 90). The Industrial Revolution that allowed for this mass production of formula also engaged more women (and sometimes children) in labor outside of the home. Jacqueline Wolf noted that in the late nineteenth century, working-class women increasingly left their infants at home "with grade school daughters and artificial food" (2003: 2001).

The commercial production of baby food also contributed to the decreasing length of time babies were nursed from the breast/chest. As Amy Bentley noted in a historical analysis of infant food and feeding in the United States:

> [i]n the space of a few decades (from the late-nineteenth to the mid-twentieth centuries) mainstream advice regarding infant feeding, and also to a great extent

practice, changed from near-exclusive consumption of breast milk (whether from the mother or from a wet nurse) and the introduction of solids later in the infant's first year, to bottle-feeding and the introduction of solids at six-weeks postpartum. Although mothers and health professionals alike welcomed commercially mass-produced baby food as a convenient, affordable way to provide more fruits and vegetables year-round for American babies, the creation and marketing of Gerber baby food, which from its inception dominated the US market, helped spur the introduction of solid foods into babies' diets at earlier and earlier ages. The post-World War II baby boom was the apex of this phenomenon. Industrial baby food thus functioned not only as a supplement to, but also as a substitute for, breast milk, playing an important role in the dramatic decline of breastfeeding in the twentieth century. (2006: 65)

Both the formula and baby food industries' suggestion that human breast milk is "not enough" contributed to explanatory models about breast milk's "value" beyond infancy. Formula marketing strategies from the early twentieth century contributed to the idea that prolonged nursing was not only not necessary but potentially harmful. For example, a Nestlé ad placed in *Good Housekeeping* from 1911 includes, in large and bold text, the sentence, "Don't Wait Too Long to Wean your Baby," followed by:

If you do, the little one is likely to be weak and anemic. Mother's milk is, of course, the best food for young babies, but the time comes when it isn't sufficient for the fast-growing body. (Image of advertisement in Tomori 2021: Online)

Law professor Andrea Freeman, in her book, *Skimmed: Breastfeeding, Race, and Injustice* (2020), gave the additional context of how marketing campaigns for another US-based company (PET Milk) specifically targeted Black consumers in the mid-twentieth century and in the decades that followed. Freeman detailed how PET capitalized on the birth of Black quadruplets in North Carolina in the 1940s (the Fultz sisters); their images were used in advertisements as they grew to illustrate the benefits of formula to grow healthy children (Freeman 2020).

In part due to these marketing campaigns, a common explanatory model (often discussed in online support groups as something EN parents hear from others, including healthcare professionals) has emerged suggesting there is no nutritional value in breast milk for children beyond the infant stage—that after infancy, chest/breastfeeding is purely about bonding or comfort (for parents and/or children), as if at a certain point, breast milk "magically" becomes "like water" or loses any nutritive value. Although breast milk becomes less important as a source of calories as a child gets older and eats solid foods, it does not cease to be a source of nutrients and immunoglobulins. Breast milk does vary in composition over time in fascinating ways though. The early milk (colostrum) produced during the first few days after childbirth functions more to create the microbiome of the child (or children, in the case of multiples) than it does to feed the child (Gopalakrishna and Hand 2020). In a comparative study of the breast milk of *Mam*-Maya Guatemalan mothers, Gonzalez et al. (2021) found a significantly different set of bacterial species present in the milk of mothers in "early" versus "late" stage lactation, although late was defined as 109–184 days post-partum, so EN as defined in this book was not captured. The authors mention that some of the bacteria in late stage lactation have a role in "bioremediation," or the breaking down of environmental pollutants in the body. Czosnykowska-Łukacka et al. (2018) conducted one of only a small number of studies on breast milk produced beyond the infant stage; they analyzed breast milk for up to four years of lactation and found that the macronutrient (carbohydrates, fats, and proteins) ratio changed significantly over time, with the concentration of fat and protein being higher in milk produced later in lactation, presumably as the milk production adapts to meet the needs of children at different stages of development.

Yet another issue that has affected how people of all backgrounds and social classes have come to think about public chest/breastfeeding and about EN has to do with the increased sexualization of women's breasts since the mid-twentieth century, particularly in the years after the Second World War. While nipples are erogenous zones for people of all gender identities, the perception that breasts, in particular voluptuous breasts, are constructed as a central feature of feminine sexuality and attractiveness has not always existed and does not exist in the same way cross-culturally. In an article about changing attitudes about the feminine breast in the United States, Coleman (2021) described the complex factors that served to shift public perception of women's breasts to be a symbol of "sex appeal, not maternity" (Coleman 2021: 10). These included the role of the film and fashion industry in redefining women as less capable and more in need of men (a reactionary response to the increased number of women in the workforce during the Second World War) and large breasts as representing the abundance of the post-war era.

Zaikman and Houlihan (2022) conducted a survey with over 500 online participants in the United States in 2018 on perceptions of breast exposure and public nursing. The three factors they found to be most associated with negative attitudes about public nursing were the hypersexualization of the breast, "sexist attitudes," and a lack of familiarity with chest/breastfeeding (2022: 24), and they make a case for how the latter (lack of familiarity and knowledge about chest/breastfeeding) fuels sexist attitudes. They use the term "erotophobic" to refer to fears about the potentially erotic nature of a child nursing from the breast. One of my in-depth interviewees, Nia, who was twenty-eight at the time of our interview, identified as Black/African American and had a Master's degree in a social science field; she also worked as a doula and became an IBCLC (International Board Certified Lactation Consultant) after her son was weaned, and she mentioned that while she did not have any issues personally with breasts serving to feed her child, some of her friends did, to the point where they did not want to nurse their babies from the body at all. She said,

> Even though I'm a whole lactation consultant, it's kind of stigmatized for them—seeing the breast as just sexual. And [they were] not wanting to attach their baby; they're more willing to pump, but not necessarily wanting to put baby to breast.

When a child is perceived as more mature (because they can walk and talk, for example), erotophobia surrounding feeding from one's body seems to increase, primarily for others, but sometimes for those who are practicing EN themselves, manifesting in nursing aversion, which will be discussed more in Chapter 7. I identified a common theme in the language that some people (from strangers to partners) use when making a comment that it was time to wean a child. Often these comments came from masculine-presenting or cis-het males, who were more likely than people of other identities to use more vulgar terms in relation to the breast or the act of nursing when they felt that this nursing relationship should come to an end. This could be understood as a kind of "hostile sexism," which Zaikman and Houlihan (2022: 25) mentioned in relation to attitudes about nursing, citing Glick and Fiske's (1996) description of this term.

Later in the twentieth century, in both the United States and globally, advertisements for formula referenced second wave feminism and the ability of women to work outside of the home if they were free from the burdens of prolonged nursing. In contemporary contexts, this trope of chest/breastfeeding and EN in particular as uncompensated time and physical and emotional labor that primarily impacts women emerges frequently in media and feminist discourse. EN does involve a significant expenditure of time and physical labor from lactating parents, but it can be argued that formula feeding does as well. Anthropologist Maxine Margolis, in *Mothers and Such: Views of Women and How They Have Changed* (1984), theorized that the introduction of new technologies (labor-saving devices like dishwashers and washing machines) resulted in the increased need for women to work outside of the home so that families could in turn pay for these devices. The same might be argued for the additional costs required for purchasing formula, bottles, and breast pumps, and for paying for childcare. The ability to work outside of the home for many is as much about gender equity as it is about income, but I think it is also useful to consider how its development and promotion served capitalist goals as both a multi-billion dollar industry and as a means to allow more parents to work longer hours away from their children.[3]

Medical and public/global health authorities began to promote chest/breastfeeding again in the 1970s, particularly as formula and preparation of formula in parts of the world where access to clean water was limited caused an increase in infant mortality (Sasson 2016), and today chest/breastfeeding is strongly encouraged by the WHO, the CDC, and the AAP. However, generations of children, particularly in the United States, grew up rarely seeing or being exposed to nursing. This can also have an impact on family support. Brandice Evans (2017), in a study of nursing moms in Georgia, found that a reported source of stress was not having any family members who had experienced chest/breastfeeding. Lack of exposure to chest/breastfeeding in their families was also a common reason and predictor of whether African American participants in focus groups in DeVane-Johnson et al.'s study used formula or formula supplementation:

> One participant in the 18–29 age artificial supplementation-feeding group shared that it was a given in their family that bottle feeding was the only option, "bottles were just natural" and no conversations were needed. (2018: 76)

Even though today more than 80 percent of infants in the United States are now breastfed for some length of time, that number drops to less than 60 percent at six months and about 35 percent at one year (CDC 2022), and of course these percentages vary greatly depending on region and state; statistics beyond that are not currently collected by the CDC. In part because of this disconnect from chest/breastfeeding, seeing a child who is breastfed beyond infancy is still unusual.

Since the movement back toward encouraging exclusive nursing for infants, public health campaigns designed around the idea that "breast is best" have generated stigma toward those who do not or could not chest/breastfeed their children. Karla Knutson (2023) noted that this campaign has been fairly successful in the United States in terms of increasing the number of children who receive breast milk for some amount of time, but the underlying "lactivist" ideology of "Breast is Best," she wrote,

> functions as a normative system to monitor and discipline women who act "out of bounds" by not abiding by the rhetoric of "breast is best"—whether by not breastfeeding or by not breastfeeding for the length of time recommended by leading medical organizations. (2023: 113)

There has been a backlash against this "breast is best" ideology that, in turn, affects some parents who practice EN. The backlash is a reaction to the idea, perpetuated by the media and within the medical community, that equates nursing with "good" mothering or parenting. The resentment many parents feel about the pressure to initiate and maintain chest/breastfeeding in a country where so little support is typically offered can result in a perception that the practice of EN itself is a form of judgment about their parenting, and this in turn creates additional stigma for some who practice EN. As will be discussed in future chapters, however, most people who practice EN did not necessarily plan it—and they may have gone into their nursing journey with their own prejudices about the strangeness of nursing a child who can walk and talk.

The Future of EN Stigma

In the contemporary context, both public chest/breastfeeding of children of any age and nursing beyond infancy are still stigmatized and are generally seen as practices that are "out of place," and thus subject to stigma. Chest/breastfeeding in the popular imagination has come to be associated mainly with infancy and invisibility, so the idea of continuing to nurse into childhood can blur and confound popular understandings of the borders and boundaries of child development and create moral panic about a child's future independence and productivity. In this chapter, I have discussed some of the origins of the contemporary taboos related to EN in the United States, including the roles of the formula and baby food industry and the ever-increasing emphasis on putting people to "work" that ultimately benefits the wealthiest in a stratified economy. As we enter the second quarter of the twenty-first century, lower fertility rates are increasingly becoming a political topic in the United States and other nations where there is growing rhetoric and panic over the alleged consequences of depopulation to the global economy. At present, however, new parents (particularly among the working class) are pressured to return to work as soon as possible after childbirth, thus making it unlikely that EN will become a common-enough practice that stigma associated with this practice will dissipate significantly, though social media may play a part in allowing people to be more open about this practice. In the next chapter, I include an overview of weaning practices cross-culturally and across species, primarily to explore and critique ideas about this practice as either natural versus unnatural, typical versus atypical, or normal versus abnormal in humans.

3

"Nature" and Culture in Extended Nursing

A narrative that circulates frequently on EN support groups online is by freelance writer Ruth Kamnitzer (2009), originally from Canada, who wrote about her experience living in Mongolia when she accompanied her husband on a research trip. She commented on the vastly different parenting practices she observed there, including parenting in early infancy to weaning. She noted the difference in what was discussed as "normal" in these two cultural contexts:

> In my prenatal class in small-town Canada, where Calum [her son] was born, breast feeding had been introduced with a video showing a particularly sporty-looking Swedish mother breast feeding her toddler while out skiing. A shudder ran through the group: "Sure, it's great for babies, but by the time they're walking and talking . . . ?" That was pretty much the consensus. I kept my counsel. It was my turn to be surprised when one of my new Mongolian friends told me she had breastfed until she was nine years old. I was so jaw-dropped flabbergasted that at first I dismissed it as a joke. Considering my son weaned just after turning four, I'm now a little embarrassed about my adamant disbelief. While nine years is pretty old to be breast feeding, even by Mongolian standards, it's not actually off the scale.

Although she noted that most children self-wean or are pressured by other kids to wean before age four in Mongolia, the degree to which public chest/breastfeeding and discussions of nursing and breast milk were normalized in Mongolia provided her with an "entirely different vision of how it all could be" (Kamnitzer 2009: Online), a phrase that illustrates how living in another culture different from your own can transform your worldview. I remember reading this essay and reflecting on stories in the Western media of children in the United States or United Kingdom who were still nursing occasionally when they were eight, nine, or older. I realized that I had my own biases in thinking that these were simply examples of sensationalistic journalism. Nursing children as old as portrayed in these stories seemed too long and strange to me, but after both my own experience with EN and reading about the experiences of others cross-culturally, it did not seem outside the realm of possibility that my son could have kept going with nursing well beyond age five. I also noticed in comments where others had posted Kamnitzer's story online, it was often in response to parents who were concerned that there could be long-term consequences because their child had not self-weaned, and this story was intended to be reassuring to them.

Kamnitzer's story about the normalcy of EN in Mongolia recalls something that anthropologist Margaret Mead said about her fieldwork in Samoa. The documentary *Margaret Mead: An Observer Observed* (Yans-McLaughlin and Seidman 1996) features clips and interviews from different times in her life. In one interview excerpt, she talks about her research on adolescence in American Samoa in the 1920s, which suggested a cultural, or at least biocultural, rather than purely hormonal or biological explanation for adolescent angst. She said:

> I didn't know at that point, you know, whether there'd be twenty primitive[1] societies or 200, [that] would show the same thing or not. In anthropology, you only have to show once that it's possible for a culture to make, say, a period of life easy where it's hard everywhere else . . . in order to [make] a major point that if any society can have institutions and arrangements that make it easy to grow up, then it isn't biologically given that you have to have a terrible time. And that was the principal point that I made when I wrote *Coming of Age in Samoa.*

For me, although establishing nursing turned out to be extremely difficult, after about a month and for the next several years, I sought parenting choices related to infant and child feeding that made things as easy as possible for myself. I enjoyed being "free" (in my perception) to not have to sterilize bottles or purchase formula, and I enjoyed being able to provide milk when my son was sick or hurt, both sentiments repeated by many of my interlocutors. I felt like the challenges of EN could have been minimized with different societal attitudes and support structures. I also wanted the validation that EN was not harmful to my child in the short or long term, and at that time (2007–12), I had not yet found online support groups. Part of the validation for me came from looking to other cultures—following Mead, I felt that if there were other societies (or even just one) where EN and child-led weaning were practiced and where it did not negatively impact child development, it is not a "given" that EN is harmful or abnormal.

In Chapter 2, I attempted to demonstrate how and why EN in particular came to seem strange and out of place in the United States (and elsewhere). Although

Kamintzer's story above and other examples I give in this chapter show that EN is not considered to be "abnormal" or "unnatural" in all societies, does this mean that EN and child-led weaning are more "natural" and "normal" practices than other feeding/weaning strategies? Is it possible, as some anthropologists and others have suggested, to say there is a "natural" age when child-led weaning would or should take place?

Some of my interlocutors did assume that EN and related parenting practices are "obviously" the most natural because of what they had heard or read about what our hominid ancestors, nonhuman primate relatives, and contemporary foraging societies did or do, but the notion of any purely natural practice for humans, as beings who are heavily influenced by culture and environment, is a complicated one and generally flawed. With this chapter, I wanted to provide a critical discussion of problems involved in trying to describe these practices as either "the most natural" for humans or as "abnormal" and "unnatural." The many complicated cultural, environmental, political, and economic factors that affect the experience of infant/child feeding and weaning and that impact growth and emotional and physiological development later in life make it difficult to say that any strategy is "best" or even "optimal" for all children or families.

Deconstructing "Nature" versus "Un-Nature"

Human milk is of course a substance produced by the human body with components that are known to be vital and beneficial for infant growth and development, and there are numerous studies that link chest/breastfeeding to better health outcomes for both the lactating parent and child (Bartick et al. 2017). Still, children can also survive and thrive despite not being exclusively or ever breastfed. In her book, *Is Breast Best?*, Joan Wolf (2011) has revisited some of the studies that claim to demonstrate long-term "better" outcomes in terms of social, emotional, and physical health and even intellectual development and "intelligence":

> When researchers consistently eliminate the explanatory power of potentially significant variables, including behavior, through inadequate controls, faulty conclusions become operating assumptions. (2011: 37)

Wolf suggested there are too many confounding factors to conclude that chest/breastfeeding will necessarily lead to better long-term outcomes for children than formula feeding.

Biological anthropologist Jonathan Marks has argued that the attempt to define human nature and to specify what is natural versus unnatural for humans by comparing practices across cultures or across species results in something of a futile task:

> To define human nature is to define as well human un-nature. If carnivory shaped our evolution, as one sociobiologist has written, then being a vegetarian is unnatural. And yet people survive, and thrive, and quite happily, as vegetarians. If polygyny is human nature, then monogamous people are unnatural—and yet many are happy that way. Human nature is merely the range of things humans are capable of. Some are noble, some are destructive, most are merely variants. But if humans can be found to be both peaceful and aggressive, say, then it makes little sense to speak of one or the other as being human nature—and it's a ridiculously trivial observation to say that both are human nature. That is because the question is framed archaically. Nature and culture act as a synergy. If the human is like a cake, culture is like the eggs, not like the icing; it is an inseparable part, not a superficial glaze. Whatever humans do, or look like, is a product of both. (Marks 2003: 176-7)

Marks has pointed out that even the inclusion of nursing as a defining criterion for the class Mammalia in the taxonomic system has a cultural and political origin (Marks 2003: 50), and while it is not that nursing is "not natural," it is difficult to say that a single modality of feeding (or weaning) infants and young children is "natural to mammals" when the category of animal classification used to define mammals was itself strongly shaped by culture and history. Marks has also noted that assuming that the idea that nonhuman primate behavior can be "illuminating for human nature" can also be understood as a "naturalistic fallacy" (2003: 161) particularly since, despite the fact that we share a common ancestor, evolutionary divergence took place millions of years ago. The suggestion that EN is a purely "natural" practice because it was standard throughout much of hominid prehistory or because it is practiced in foraging societies today or in some nonhuman primate species may also lend itself to the perception that it is a more "animalistic" or "primitive" practice and that, from a cultural evolutionary perspective, people in more "developed countries" no longer need to practice it.

Virginia Thorley, an Australian historian who also trained as a lactation consultant and served in international organizations related to chest/breastfeeding support, has written about the problematic aspects of calling chest/breastfeeding the "normal" way to feed infants and the "only" way that humans fed infants before formula was invented. There are examples of regions where, centuries before the introduction of commercial formula, nursing of infants had come to be of very short duration or virtually "abandoned" as a practice in favor of alternative forms of feeding, and nursing was highly discouraged by physicians in Western Europe in the Late Middle Ages and beyond. She noted that in seventeenth- and eighteenth-century Iceland, cow's milk and pre-chewed fish were given to infants very early on, and only the most impoverished families resorted to chest/breastfeeding (2019: 40). Often the choice to not breastfeed at all was not out of necessity but a choice based on the prestige of feeding from local milk-producing livestock that were part of community identity. Citing the work of Garðarsdóttir (2002) and Hastrup (1992), Thorley wrote:

> Women believed that doing the best for their babies meant feeding them on the more highly regarded and economically valued cow's milk from their dairies in preference to human milk that had no monetary value and was considered unhealthy. (2019: 40)

Although Thorley, as a lifetime advocate for chest/breastfeeding, has written that breast milk is "superior" to formula in helping to build "the infant gut biome and maintaining immune homeostasis beyond weaning" (2019: 39), she suggested it is better to refer to "breastfeeding as 'biologically normal' or 'physiologically normal', acknowledging that it is not necessarily normal to a culture" (2019: 43).

Considering the above insights, I wondered if it was even useful to this book to describe different nursing and weaning practices in other species or in other cultures, since these practices should not dictate what parents do in terms of feeding their children. After conducting in-depth interviews with twelve couples over time who had planned and attempted chest/breastfeeding their children, Laura Fitzwater Gonzales found that

> when breastfeeding is perceived as natural, it negatively affects the identities of mothers who struggle to breastfeed, and it also discourages mothers who struggle from seeking out breastfeeding support. (2018: 212)

However, the phenomenon of lactating humans and other species producing milk from their bodies exists across time and space, and a comparison of practices is both interesting and revealing, not in terms of what is "the most natural" but mostly in terms of the ways that complex circumstances affect nursing duration and weaning. I also thought that it was important to touch on the wide variation in these practices as well as to contrast with some of the popular beliefs about either the essential "naturalness" or "strangeness" of both EN and child-led weaning. I think there is value in showing that EN and associated practices (on-demand nursing, co-sleeping, alloparental care, and child-led/offspring-led or gentle weaning) exist in both contemporary and historical contexts in human societies around the world and among our closest primate relatives, and that some parenting strategies (and the support systems or structures to carry them out) can make life easier for parents and children today. This information is valuable to and often shared by parents and caregivers in online spaces who practice EN in the United States, as it reassures them that their choices will not be causing irreparable damage to their children. Below, I highlight some of the anthropological research that has been conducted on nursing initiation, EN, and weaning among nonhuman primates and in different cultures.

Barriers and Facilitators of Nursing Initiation

For many adult humans, initiating chest/breastfeeding does not come easily or "naturally"; it is often a learning process for both the lactating caregiver and the infant. In humans and nonhuman primates, instinct and "hormones appear to play a much smaller role in the initiation and maintenance of primate maternal behavior" than in other mammals (Nicolson 1991: 26), suggesting that the social environment and learning play an important role in parenting for primates. Primate is the "order" in the taxonomic system that we share with apes, monkeys, tarsiers, lemurs, many other smaller nonhuman primate species, and with our hominid ancestors. One of the characteristics of members of this order is that offspring require prolonged care from adults (relative to other species) before they can care for themselves and survive on their "own," though most continue to live in social groups. Nonhuman primates in captivity who were raised individually or separated early from their mothers demonstrate lower levels of skill in terms of maternal care (e.g., nursing, correct holds of infants), though sometimes these skills improved with subsequent births (Nicolson 1991; Volk 2009). Nonhuman primates raised in captivity and isolated from others do not automatically know how to nurse their offspring, which suggests that nursing behaviors are also not exclusively about instinct for our nonhuman primate relatives, even if there are "typical" practices in the wild (Volk 2009). There was a news story that circulated in 2023 about an orangutan mother at the Richmond Zoo (in North Carolina) who had herself been orphaned at nine months and for whom nursing and caring for an infant did not come "naturally." Her first infant was hand-raised by zookeepers because she could not nurse and did not know how to care for it. When she was pregnant with her second baby, she was shown videos of orangutan mothers giving birth and caring for their young in the months leading up to the birth of her own baby, and the lead zookeeper gave demonstrations using a stuffed baby orangutan. Another zookeeper, Whitlee Turner, who was nursing her own infant, spent time demonstrating nursing to the orangutan mother. Within a day of the zookeeper's demonstration with her human baby, Zoe started to nurse her own infant (Blair 2023), which suggests the importance of teaching and learning in infant feeding for some nonhuman primates.

For humans, a lack of ongoing lactation support and family support can be a factor in problems with nursing initiation and with early weaning. Some human infants latch well right away, but many do not, and even for those who do, the lactating parent generally has to learn different holds and positions that make chest/breastfeeding possible. In families, cultures, and societies where nursing is more visible and shared caregiving ("alloparenting") of parents and non-biological parents, in roles that include holding others' babies or nursing another person's child, are a part of everyday life, there may be less active learning involved and more unconscious learning, so that in such societies, chest/breastfeeding and EN might seem less "out of place." Anthropologist Frank L'Engle Williams (2020) has discussed the important role of alloparental care from fathers in infant and early childhood care throughout human evolution and in contemporary foraging societies. Barry Hewlett and Steve Winn (2014) noted the role of allomaternal nursing and allomaternal care (care for children by other family or community members) among Aka foragers in the Central African Rainforest; among the Aka, grandmothers and fathers were active in both childcare and allowing children to either nurse or latch on to their nipples for comfort.

Based on research with the indigenous K'exel Maya in Guatemala (whose subsistence is based primarily on small-scale agriculture), Chary et al. (2011: 178) gave an example of how alloparenting played a part in a solution to a nursing strike in an infant that was believed to be caused by a culture-bound syndrome known as *empacho*. The mother "thought the '*tres leches*' (three milks) remedy" could cure her son. "She would have to find three other mothers to wet nurse, and only then would he accept her breast again." This type of solution to a problem with nursing is less common or accessible in the United States, though there are parents in United States contexts who find and seek out similar support when they are having trouble maintaining their milk supply or getting an infant to continue to nurse (Wilson 2018).

Most of my in-depth interviewees discussed challenges they faced with nursing initiation with one or more of their children. In addition to lack of lived experience with nursing or holding infants, initiation of nursing can also be complicated by a variety of factors related to birth circumstances and the health of the parent and infant post-partum. Melissa, a white woman who was forty-seven at the time of our interview and who had practiced EN with four children, described how her experiences establishing nursing were challenging with both her first and fourth child. With her first (born in 2007), she had an infection "that manifested itself during labor," resulting in her newborn being put into a "special care nursery":

> I got to hold her a little bit right after she was born and to try to nurse her, but neither one of us knew what we were doing, so we didn't get far. Then they took her, and I didn't get to see her again for several hours because it took a long time for my epidural to wear off, and I was also being treated and tested for the infection. When I was finally able to be wheeled down to see her, the nurse on duty asked if I had fed the baby, and I told her, "I tried, but she didn't get it." The nurse said, "well, if she doesn't 'get it,' we'll have to give her formula, because she needs to eat." That of course seemed very disheartening, because I was trying to do all the things I had read you're supposed to do to prevent nipple confusion. Luckily, that nurse's shift ended soon after that, and the next one seemed much more in line with my way of thinking; she said that babies aren't born hungry, and it's ok if they don't get much milk at first. Our hospital stay was extended because of my fever, and there was one instance where someone gave her a pacifier against my explicit wishes. It was like some of the nurses just didn't care about my efforts to establish a breastfeeding relationship, or they thought that was pointless, or maybe they just didn't think about it at all. Then some of the other nurses were really supportive and understood what I was trying to do and didn't pressure me about anything. And not long after getting home, my baby and I got the hang of breastfeeding, and we had a very good, two-and-a-half year breastfeeding relationship.

When Melissa's infant didn't "get it," the first nurse's solution was for her to move to formula. Though an infant receiving formula from a bottle does not have to signal the end of the nursing relationship, it can make it more difficult to establish (LLL International 2024b). Melissa's third child was born in 2018, and their nursing journey was initially complicated by the fact that her newborn son had respiratory issues and had to be transported to a NICU at a different hospital than where they gave birth. She described a much more supportive experience at the hospital related to supporting chest/breastfeeding, which might reflect changes taking place in the decade between these children's births:

> While I had to stay at [the hospital where I gave birth] the first night, the folks at [the hospital where my son was] called me to ask for permission to feed [my son] donor breast milk. I could not believe that but was so impressed! So of course I said yes. I think they also asked if he could have a pacifier, and my own opinion on those had changed, so I didn't mind, especially since I couldn't be with him. And [the hospital] provided me with a pump so I could try to get the colostrum going. Even though I only got a tiny quantity, the nurses said how great it was that I was able to do that, and somehow [my son] got it. I can't remember how . . . So he had bottles in the NICU, but only breast milk, either mine or the donor milk. I think I was also able to breastfeed him there, but it was a little different because of the NICU situation. There was just a really strong emphasis on breastfeeding and breast milk. And he got to go home after another day. We did supplement with formula at home, but only for a couple of days, because he had been on bottles and we thought maybe he was already accustomed to the larger quantities you can get from a bottle vs the probably smaller quantities you'd get just from colostrum while breastfeeding directly from the start. We quit the bottles as soon as my milk supply came in, which has never been later than day five for me. I think he hurt the most of all my babies at the beginning of nursing, and I used nipple shields [which help with latching in some cases] for a while. He's the only baby I used them with. Those were so helpful. But before too long, we established a very good and long lasting breastfeeding relationship.

Melissa's narrative is illustrative of the experiences of many parents in the United States who deliver in hospital settings; even in her more recent example of receiving support from hospital staff, it is clear that there are so many factors involved in being able to begin and ultimately establish "a long lasting breastfeeding relationship" in situations where there are any complications associated with birth.

In my own experience, I went into parenthood feeling strongly that I wanted to exclusively nurse and have a an unmedicated birth, which I thought would facilitate nursing. My son was born a few weeks premature, and a variety of circumstances associated with labor and delivery (including placenta accreta, in which the placenta did not deliver normally) prompted a round of antibiotics for both of us in the first forty-eight hours of his life. I pumped milk, and we bottle-fed for the first several days. I was fortunate enough to be allowed to remain in the hospital, where I also had an opportunity to work briefly with a lactation consultant, though our interactions were less than an hour total in the five days we spent at the hospital. My newborn still developed jaundice that comes from hyperbilirubinemia, elevated bilirubin levels that are common in preterm infants and affect "approximately 60 percent of fullterm neonates" (Clements 2013: Online). Jaundice can develop from a variety of causes (including mother and infant having a different blood type, as was true for us), but it is sometimes associated with infants not getting enough milk through exclusive chest/breastfeeding. According to Clements (2013: Online) in an article for Duke Health,

> although breastfeeding is also considered a risk factor, it is actually *lack of effective breastfeeding* that is the risk factor. The likelihood of problems with nursing are minimized by nursing the newborn as soon after birth as possible and to continue nursing eight to twelve times per day for the first several days. Breast milk is an ideal food for babies, and jaundice is usually not a reason to add formula to the diet.

In hospital settings, hyperbilirubinemia often results in healthcare professionals urging parents to supplement with formula unless donor milk is available, as Melissa mentioned. In our case, in addition to phototherapy, the hospital strongly urged supplementing with formula, which we resisted at first but wound up doing for several feedings while in the hospital, and my son's bilirubin levels improved. Once we were allowed to go home, I was able to exclusively give breast milk, first through a combination of pumping/bottle feeding and later through nursing only. I was somewhat resentful of the hospital staff and felt pressured to use formula as a supplement during this first week of my baby's life, but I did not feel like I had the knowledge or authority to contest it at the time. We were also sent home with a supply of formula and encouraged to use it. Although the focus of this book is not on the initiation of chest/breastfeeding, these early experiences with nursing play an important role in why many people do not continue nursing their infants beyond a few weeks.

Nursing Duration in Nonhuman Primates and People

In support groups for EN online, and among my in-depth interviewees, parents and other caregivers of children put varying degrees of thought and effort into creating a plan for nursing and less into planning for weaning. Some aim to nurse for as long as feasibly possible given their work situation and other limitations. For those who planned on child-led weaning, the duration often far exceeded the amount of time they had planned to nurse. Some planned to child-led wean but found themselves needing to make a choice at some point about weaning because of a variety of factors, such as problems with milk production, a child or parent's health issue, work, travel, divorce, another pregnancy, aversion, or just feeling "ready" to be done. Others planned to actively wean earlier but wound up continuing to nurse through some of these events.

Michelle, a white physician and researcher who was forty-seven at the time of our virtual interview, talked about a time early on in her nursing journey in which she had to decide whether or not to continue nursing or switch to formula. Her son latched well initially:

> I mean, it was hard because of the physical stuff and the pain and everything, but in terms of like, he latched, he ate, and you know, like I didn't have that early difficulty that I know so many people have.

But, she said:

> I don't remember making a conscious decision about it until I started like having supply issues and had to make the decision, like, "No, I want to commit to breast milk only and not do formula." I think that was like, that felt like the first branch point, but I didn't hit that branch point until he was probably, like, two months old.

This concept of a "branch point" is a useful one for conceptualizing when and how lactating parents arrive at different places with nursing or weaning. These branch points could come at different times and from different circumstances (e.g., a pregnancy or an illness), in which the parent has to take a more active role in decision-making about either abrupt weaning or "gentle weaning," another practice that involves intentional practices on the part of the parent to wean but avoids abrupt refusal of chest/breastfeeding on the part of the parent and opts for a more gradual approach to prepare a child emotionally for the end of the chest/breastfeeding relationship, and some parents wind up tandem nursing, or nursing more than one child. Caitlyn, a white woman who was thirty-six at the time of our interview, said that her difficult childbirth experience (which included an unplanned C-section) in the hospital impacted her decision to continue nursing for as long as her daughter wanted to nurse, "Everything in parenting—I wanted to do it, I guess, 'naturally' is the word and just as biologically normal as I possibly can," though this did not pan out in practice. Her early experiences with nursing were also "really terrible," but eventually they established a "really good rhythm." She said, "I was like, I'm not stopping her. I'm going to let her dictate how this goes, and I'm open to that." Her child continued to nurse for three and a half years, and weaning was "mostly child-led." Caitlyn was pregnant at the time of the interview and planned to nurse her second child for "as long or longer."

When I asked Stephanie, a white woman who worked in public health (age thirty-two at the time of our interview) about parenting strategies, she said she did not plan much beyond aiming to breastfeed:

> I feel like in preparing to be a parent, I really focused a lot on labor and delivery, and I didn't think about anything beyond that, so I've kind of just been taking things as they come at me, so I don't think I was even aware that there were parenting styles until you know, really, more so thinking about as my child got older and there were behavioral issues . . . I realized that there were different kinds of philosophies. I knew in my mind that one year was a goal because I'd heard that that was a goal in the US or whatever . . . but then I also heard the worldwide average was four years or whatever, [but] I didn't think about actively weaning him. I thought he would just magically stop at one year.

When I asked if she had expected to still be nursing past two years, she said, "it never occurred to me."

The idea of a worldwide average for weaning that Stephanie mentioned is something that is often repeated on extended nursing support groups as not only a goal but as an explanation for why EN and child-led weaning is "normal" and "natural." These "averages" often appear on websites and in popular discourse on weaning, and I have noticed they are a useful tool for some EN parents as a counter to the idea that their child is "too old" to be nursing, but the figure itself is not a mathematically accurate representation. In 2009, on her website, anthropologist Katherine Dettwyler critiqued the figure of a global "average" of 4.2 years for weaning cross-culturally, which she noted was published in Ruth Lawrence's book, *Breastfeeding: A Guide for the Medical Profession* (1994: 312). Dettwyler wrote:

> What would a world-wide average really mean? How would one even calculate such a thing as a single, worldwide, average age for cessation of breastfeeding? Take each child's age at weaning and add them up and divide them by the

number of children? Do you add together and then divide by all the published figures for each "culture," so that my study of 116 Bambara [referring to her fieldwork among the Bambara of Mali] children from a peri-urban community counts as one data point, and someone else's study of a rural Bambara village counts as another data point? Or do you average the two averages, and report only one figure for each culture? Or do you take an average age at weaning for each country, based on all the studies done on various ethnic groups within that geopolitical entity? In that case, the millions of children in China count for one data point, the same as the thousands in Mali. (Dettwyler 2009: Online)

Though calculating an "average" does not make sense, a broad range of weaning times can be observed cross-culturally and medians can be calculated within single cultures given enough data. Dettwyler analyzed data collected by twentieth-century ethnographers in places where infant formula had not yet been introduced, that this "literature is fairly consistent in reporting that children are often weaned between two and five years of age across a wide variety of traditional societies" (1995: 43). Anthropologist Patricia Stuart-Macadam (1995: 84), writing about nursing in prehistory, cites examples from other researchers' work on nursing duration cross-culturally that include reports of weaning in different societies up to age seven, with this higher number based on her own research in Inuit communities (1995: 84).

Dettwyler has pointed out that many of the early ethnographers were not focusing on chest/breastfeeding specifically or doing systematic studies and in some cases their data may represent "ideals or cultural norms" (1995: 43), which means that in practice, weaning could take place much earlier or later than reported. More recently, ethnographers have done more systematic research on nursing and weaning behaviors in foraging societies, including research conducted by biological anthropologists Melvin Konner and Marjorie Shostak on the foraging society, the !Kung San (who live in the Kalahari Desert in southern Africa), which produced more nuanced data on weaning, demonstrating that not all children in a single society are weaned at the same time; they also observed changes in typical weaning duration over time. In Konner and Shostak's research among this group in 1970, they observed that children were weaned between ages three and four in 1970, with some children nursing beyond four years, whereas in 1975, "the modal age was two to three years, with no children nursing beyond four years" (Konner and Shostak 1987: 12), which could reflect societal changes during this interval.

Duration of nursing in foraging and other small-scale or traditional societies cannot help us determine what is a "normal" age for weaning, but this data does point to the fact that what is considered "extended" nursing in the United States is, or has been, considered "normal" or "typical" in other societies. However, because of the highly variable cultural and environmental influences on human societies, Katherine Dettwyler has suggested it is useful to look to our closest relatives in the animal kingdom to get a better understanding of what might be "normal" for humans if certain cultural restrictions or economic systems were not factors and if weaning were based "on purely physiological considerations" (1995: 39), though this assumes that nonhuman primates are not also subject to external influences (including culture/learned behaviors and environmental degradation). She collected and analyzed information on typical weaning times for nonhuman primates (Dettwyler 2004, 1995) with the goal of extrapolating an estimate of a natural duration of nursing among humans from an evolutionary or biological/physiological perspective (1995: 39). The task itself of suggesting nonhuman primate weaning as a proxy for human weaning could be critiqued as a form of naturalistic fallacy, as discussed above, but she does acknowledge the many cultural factors that impact nursing among humans and "make human societies unique and varied." Dettwyler has written "predictions for a natural age of weaning in modern human populations, based on nonhuman primate patterns, range between 2.5 years and a maximum of seven years" (1995: 39). Her comparison of nonhuman primate weaning times shows a great deal of variation among these species, but among the great apes (gorillas, orangutans, and chimpanzees), average weaning times were four to six times the number of days of gestation (e.g., 1538 days, or over four years, for gorillas) (Dettwyler 1995: 63).

Dettwyler has also noted that the calculation of a natural weaning time in primates based on tripling or quadrupling of birth weight, or, as Charnov and Berrigan (1993) suggested, when they reach a third of their adult weight, is not useful for human populations, where there is such dramatic cultural variability in terms of diet and adult weight (Dettwyler 1995: 49). She noted that some of the literature on weaning that predated her research suggested that a natural time for weaning would match with gestation times of a species, which in humans would be just nine months, but she notes that this was based primarily on studies of smaller mammals. Dettwyler did suggest that one developmental milestone, eruption of the first permanent molar, which typically occurs around age six in humans, also corresponds to when children's immune systems reach "adult immune competence" (1995: 56), so she concluded that if there is a natural weaning age, it would probably be at least six years. Six years might seem well beyond what most Americans imagine is a "normal" duration of nursing, but it is regularly reported as an age for child-led weaning in online groups. Although Dettwyler has been an advocate for chest/breastfeeding rights and has been vocal about the benefits of EN and related parenting practices, she has also been explicit about not suggesting that all parents *must* or *should* practice EN; instead, she wanted to "establish the 'hominid blueprint' for weaning in an attempt to illuminate the mismatch between our evolutionary heritage as primates and current pediatric advice and practice in the US" (1995: 40).[2]

In both humans and nonhuman primates, weaning is never "purely physiological," as environmental stress and group-specific learned behaviors (particularly among our closest primate relatives who exhibit characteristics of what we understand as culture) may play a part in when offspring are weaned. In discussing weaning times among mammals, Dettwyler noted that it is "assumed to be primarily a function of genetics and instinct, with some environmental component related to child growth thrown in for good measure" (1995: 45), but there are some obvious ways in which humans have impacted weaning among other species with which they have had close contact for millennia. This can include prolonging lactation for domesticated mammals for milk production and abrupt, forced weaning among animals used/sold for meat or for their labor or that are considered pets. Mammals in captivity, in zoos or research labs, also experience stressors and conditions that might also impact weaning times. Environmental degradation and climate change can also impact weaning times for mammals in the wild.

Data on "typical" weaning times in mammals might be skewed by a number of factors, including environment and human actions relative to these species but also the invisibility or unrecognizability (to researchers) of nursing behaviors, individual animal temperament, and, especially in our closest primate relatives, culture/learned behaviors and agency. Smith et al. (2017) also make the important point that observations of orangutan (and presumably other great apes) weaning in the wild are particularly difficult for many reasons, including the long duration of nursing, and the fact that nursing can take place "inconspicuously," and night nursing may be common among older primate offspring. The hidden nature of much nursing activity could lead to underestimates of weaning times by primatologists who based their assessments primarily on a few observations. In addition, they note that observing orangutans with a focus on nursing and weaning can be difficult because most researchers cannot sustain years of observations. Through an analysis of barium concentrations in orangutan teeth from Borneo and Sumatra, Smith et al. (2017) identified two orangutans that had nursed for more than eight years, including one that had not yet weaned at the age of death (8.8 years).

This idea of how inconspicuous nursing behaviors can be is also relevant to the observed and reported nursing times of humans across cultures. Participant observation might allow anthropologists to have some insight into nursing practices and duration, but many older children may drink very little human milk during the day, when it is visible to observers, but still nurse to sleep. Self-reporting of weaning may also be skewed downward in societies where EN is stigmatized because parents are aware of the stigma and potential negative consequences.

While there is variation from family to family within foraging societies and in different contemporary foraging societies, depending on their circumstances, there are certain characteristics of nursing in foraging societies that make it more likely that weaning will take place later than in agricultural or industrial societies. Lactating parents in foraging societies have more close contact with their children throughout the day, so that children have frequent access to on-demand nursing, in contrast to parents who may have to be separated from their children for part of each day for work. Parenting practices that are more common in foraging, horticultural, and other small-scale societies may also facilitate nursing in both the short and long term. At the same time, even if EN is possible and encouraged within a community, not all lactating parents may feel positively about it. As mentioned above, among the K'exel Maya in Guatemala, there is community and alloparenting support for nursing initiation; there is also an expectation within the community that mothers provide intensive caregiving of children, and these expectations are reinforced by public health messages disseminated by global health organizations (Chary et al. 2011: 172). Yet prolonged nursing is particularly difficult for these women, who spend much of their lives feeding children from their bodies. In addition to the time and labor involved, there is also food scarcity in their community, which makes nursing more challenging.

In an analysis of data from the Millennium Cohort Study in the United Kingdom, Emmott and Mace (2015) found that certain types of support from fathers and grandmothers actually decreased the duration of chest/breastfeeding among mothers. Specifically, "practical" support included frequent contact, assistance with childcare, and financial support. This was a retrospective study based on quantitative data, but it raises important questions in terms of nuancing the effects of "support" on chest/breastfeeding initiation and duration. Access to frequent practical support (e.g., having someone else prepare bottles and feed the child, rock the child to sleep) could allow the nursing parent to return to work earlier and spend more time away from their child. Emmott and Mace contrast how "practical" support in stratified, industrial societies might be different from that provided in foraging societies where parents' labor does not require separation from their children.

A Variety of Weaning Practices

The duration of chest/breastfeeding and the manner in which children or other mammalian offspring are weaned (or wean themselves) are separate but related topics. Saying that a child is weaned at six months or six years tells us nothing about *how* that child was weaned. In this section, I give a few examples of weaning practices that illustrate that both abrupt or harsh weaning techniques and gentle, more child-led weaning techniques exist across species and cultures. Some of the possible reasons for different methods of weaning are also explored here.

Many infants seem to self-wean in the first year, but lactation experts consider this to be a "nursing strike," which can be "resolved," as it might be related to changes in the lactating parents' diet, forms of stress, child illness, or many other external factors (LLL International 2024b). In Coral Wayland's (2004) qualitative research in a low-income community in the state of Acre in western Brazil, mothers talked about reasons for weaning early (before six months) that implied a strong belief in the infant's agency in refusing breast milk. In the cases Wayland described, it is clear there are other factors involved (such as one mother's decision to offer water regularly to her infant), but from the perspective of the mothers interviewed, their infants preferred formula and might starve without it. Although infants could be argued to be exerting agency in rejecting nursing from the breast, it is not because they are choosing formula over breast milk but because an external factor is temporarily making bottle feeding easier or less difficult.

Child-led weaning is discussed in EN online support groups as, if not the most "natural" form of weaning, one that avoids the stress involved, for both parents and children, of abrupt weaning. When I was nursing and struggling with the question of whether my son would ever self-wean, I often assumed that without human or other external intervention, all mammals would self-wean with no caregiver intervention when they were developmentally "ready." While this may be true of some mammals, there is variation in how infants are weaned among nonhuman primates; in some species (and perhaps among some individuals within nonhuman primate groups), weaning is "gentler" and in others, lactating parents have been observed to actively reject offspring's attempts to continue nursing after a certain time. In a Nature/PBS documentary on the snub-nosed monkey in the Chinese Himalayas (Zhinong 2015), there is an interesting example of the active (and not at all gentle) weaning process for one juvenile. The mother had started to refuse to let him nurse, and the young monkey was terribly agitated at losing access to its mother's milk; the documentary narrator characterized this as a "tantrum," and at the risk of further anthropomorphizing, it did appear to be a true emotional meltdown. He jumped wildly all around and screamed (while adult monkeys ignored him completely), spun in circles while the mom pushed him away, and then collapsed to the ground with a paw across his eyes in defeat. Li et al. (2013) have reported that among snub-nosed monkeys in the wild, there is minimal rejection on the part of mothers toward nursing at twelve months but increased rejection of offsprings' attempts to nurse after that age. Weaning that involves denial of access to milk and maternal rejection has been shown to cause high levels of stress in a study of free-ranging rhesus macaques (Mandalaywala et al. 2014), which also manifests in behaviors like tantrums and distress calls. Increased stress had a physiological effect in terms of elevated cortisol levels in the offspring's feces. Mandalaywala et al. (2014) suggested that the long-term consequences of this stress could be advantageous from an evolutionary perspective, providing an increased ability to store energy reserves and withstand increased maternal rejection. It is noteworthy that the population studied was among a free-ranging population in Cayo Santiago, Puerto Rico, which is not the native habitat for macaques. Arguably, most nonhuman primates in the wild are not truly "in the wild" anywhere on earth today, in the sense that their habitat is under consistent stress from environmental degradation, and thus, any observation of contemporary nonhuman primates may not represent a "natural interaction," if such an interaction can exist.

In both nonhuman primates and humans, there is variation in weaning practices of different lactating parents and offspring/children, and there are differences in how siblings wean themselves or are more actively weaned by parents as well. Pregnancy often impacts the lactating parent's ability or willingness to continue nursing and the offspring's desire to continue, as pregnancy can affect the taste, supply, and composition of milk (Moscone and Moore 1993). Although many EN parents practice or attempt to practice tandem nursing, the youngest child/last born in a family is often nursed the longest because pregnancy does not interfere with the nursing relationship. EN might also be more prolonged for only children.

Murphy and Murphy (1974) have written that although on-demand nursing was common for children among the Mundurucú (an indigenous group in the Amazon region who practice subsistence horticulture), and children were allowed to continue nursing through their mother's next pregnancy, when a sibling is born, the child "is told, bluntly and directly, that the breast is for the new baby and is sometimes physically shoved away" (1974: 168) if they try to nurse. The Murphys' depiction of weaning at this stage is far from "gentle," and they observed that children who were abruptly weaned with the birth of a sibling exhibit "emotional squalls, temper tantrums, continual crying, moodiness, and acute manifestations of sibling rivalry" (1974: 168). They also cite Ruth Boyer's dissertation research among the Apache (1962), in which she observed "an abrupt and total displacement of maternal attention to the newborn, with similarly traumatic results for the older child" (Murphy and Murphy 1974: 169). However, they note that Boyer's research took place in the stressful environment of the reservation.

Konner and Shostak (1987) described nursing among !Kung foragers as prolonged and relatively gradual unless or until a nurisng mother became pregnant with another child. In Marjorie Shostak's well-known life history of a !Kung woman (*Nisa*, Shostak 1981), Nisa herself described weaning as a traumatic memory in her own childhood that began when her mother got pregnant with her brother. Her mother used a bitter root at first to discourage her from nursing, but Nisa would ask for milk constantly, both during her mother's pregnancy and after her brother was born; Nisa mentioned that physical punishment and some degree of psychological manipulation by her mother and other adults in her family were involved when Nisa continued to want her mother's milk after the baby was born. Shostak notes that Nisa's story of the extreme stress and hunger she experienced and the harsh treatment from her parents may not be typical among the !Kung, but she wrote that with the exception of last born children, most children do not have significant agency in deciding when to stop nursing.

The above examples are of weaning practices that contrast with the child-led or "gentle" ideal to which many EN parents aspire. However, Fouts et al.

(2001) have suggested that twentieth-century anthropological sources about weaning practices in foraging societies are based on limited examples. They note the possibility of a Eurocentric bias in ethnographers' assessments, possibly drawn from Freudian ideas about attachment, oral fixation, and independence.

> Taken together, the psychological, anthropological, and evolutionary theories have helped create the following widely endorsed beliefs or hypotheses about weaning: (1) weaning is initiated by mothers; (2) once mothers decide to stop nursing, weaning takes place within a few days; (3) mothers use specific techniques to terminate nursing quickly; (4) weaning foods (gruels and mashed foods) are essential around the time of weaning; (5) weaning is a traumatic experience that leads to temper tantrums and displays of aggression; and (6) weaning exclusively involves mothers and their offspring and leads weanlings to establish stronger relationships with other children. As indicated above, however, these hypotheses have only been loosely informed by systematic observations of human mothers weaning their children. (2001: 31)

In mixed methods research, Fouts et al. sought to "evaluate the scientific literature by examining the social and emotional context of weaning among the Bofi foragers" (2001: 31), a group who live in the Central African Republic in the Congo Basin rainforest, and they demonstrated that the above conceptions about weaning did not apply to this society. They found that when asked about weaning, mothers said that children stopped nursing when they were "big" (generally at age three or four) or when the mother became pregnant with another child. In their observations of caregiver-child interactions, they did not witness any trauma associated with weaning. All mothers interviewed "stated that children simply stop nursing" when they are ready and that mothers did not make any attempt to wean their children if they became pregnant with another child. They did not, for example, "apply hot peppers to their nipples or use other mentioned" (2001: 35) by other Bofi women who lived in village/farm settings. In a later article (Fouts et al. 2005), the same authors illustrate how their research in these two settings suggested that weaning practices reflected "cultural schemas" rather than a more biologically deterministic motive of children to maximize their survival and "reproductive success" through attempts to nurse for as long as possible (causing supposedly inevitable parent-child conflict), as previously suggested by evolutionary biologist Robert Trivers (1974). Bofi foragers' cultural schema involves egalitarianism, respect for autonomy, and giving. . . . Limited status differences exist between individuals; for example, some men and women are better hunters and some have more medical knowledge. Foragers respect personal autonomy and do not sanction each other's behavior, [while] Bofi farmer children are expected to show deference to adults, especially older men. Farmer parents value obedience and use corporal punishment and fear as tools to modify their children's behavior. (Fouts et al. 2005: 32)

Parents among Bofi foragers "did not direct weaning and viewed weaning as child-led." The authors wrote that "one mother was asked, 'When will nursing end for your son (four-year-old)?,' she laughed and said, 'Only he knows. Ask him. I cannot know how he thinks/feels'" (Fouts et al. 2005: 33). Anthropologist Bonnie Hewlett's work (2013) has also highlighted some differences between foragers (Aka) and farmers (Ngandu) in weaning practices. EN was common in both contexts, but weaning was a more active effort on the parents' part in the farming society. Nurit Bird-David (2008) also found that among Nayaka foragers in South India, a great deal of agency was attributed to children as it related to nursing. Active or "coercive" weaning of any kind on the part of parents was not practiced among this group in her observations, but children and sometimes infants were believed to actively initiate weaning. Allomaternal care was also standard among the Nakaya.

"You Only Have to Show Once That It's Possible . . ."

With this chapter, I wanted to discuss the relevancy of the concepts of "natural" versus "unnatural" child feeding and weaning practices as they apply to humans as cultural beings. The literature points to a wide range of practices related to nursing and weaning both across cultures and species. Cross-culturally and in some nonhuman primate species, prolonged nursing and gentle weaning exist as practices and there is no evidence for long-term harm to children or offspring. To revisit Margaret Mead's quotation that "[i]n anthropology, you only have to show once that it's possible for a culture to make, say, a period of life easy where it's hard everywhere else"—there are examples of societies where nursing initiation, prolonged nursing, and child-led weaning, if never truly "easy," might be made easier by certain support systems and practices, as well as different "cultural schemas."

Instead of asking whether different infant and child feeding practices are more "natural" than others, it might be more interesting to ask what environmental and socioeconomic circumstances and what "cultural schema" (Fouts et al. 2005) result in or allow for longer duration of nursing and either facilitate or hinder child-led weaning. As in some of the examples of contemporary small-scale societies demonstrate, it is important not to over-romanticize or over-generalize about chest/breastfeeding and weaning practices, but there are examples (such as among the Bofi foragers) where it seems like EN and child-led weaning are accepted as common practice and seen as a gradual and easy process for families and children. As will be explored more in subsequent chapters, among parents in online communities and among other interlocutors for this study, a variety of external factors (including support or stigma from family and friends, the topic of the next chapter) made true "child-led" weaning difficult or, in some cases, not desirable, though they practiced EN.

4

"This Is Not Your Fight!"

Input from Friends and Family

My mom said, 'this is not your fight!' And I'm like, 'fight?' I'm not fighting. I'm just trying to get a Reuben sandwich.

The above quotation is from an interview I conducted with Sam, a white, Jewish[1] woman who held a graduate degree in creative writing but who, in part because of her experiences with nursing and with EN, sought a certificate in pediatric nutrition and was working toward becoming a certified lactation consultant at the time of our interview. In this quotation, Sam was describing an interaction she had with her mother when she was going to nurse her child in a restaurant, just a few weeks postpartum. Sam practiced EN with both of her children and was nursing her three-year-old at the time of our interview. She talked about her mother's resistance to her having nursed her children at all:

> When I was nursing my first child, [her] first granddaughter, she was extremely offended. This was a complete insult to her that I was choosing to breastfeed. My daughter was also small compared to babies that my mom had had. She was a pound smaller than my mother's smallest baby. And so there was an expectation of the background baby, and now there's the belief that in the invisible breast milk, because breast milk is invisible, there [was the concern that]—"How could this possibly be enough?" She brought a scale to my house and weighed my baby . . . Not passive aggressive—that's aggressive aggressive! So she was letting me know this was not acceptable, and I was harming my baby.

This idea of the "invisibility" of breast milk intake was a theme that was noted in online spaces as well and in pediatrician office visits, where new parents are often asked to record quantities of milk a child is consuming, which is impossible if the baby is not drinking milk from a bottle but directly from the breast. Sam believed that her mother's attitudes about chest/breastfeeding stemmed from her own experiences with parenting. Sam said she and her mother were no longer in touch, and that their mom was a "difficult person" who "had a hard time in life." "We'll just leave it as a personality disorder." She felt that her mom's behavior might be an "outlier" because of serious mental health issues, but these attitudes were not unlike those of relatives that other interlocutors and people in online support groups described.

For many reasons, including the likelihood of close contact at family gatherings or in frequent visits (or in co-living situations) or through contact online or in group chats, family and close friends are often a primary source of both stigmatizing actions/attitudes and support for people who practice EN. Alicia Simpson, in an intervention study on nursing initiation that includes interviews with African American women in the Atlanta metropolitan area, found that

> Whether or not they intended to breastfeed from the start of the study, the majority of the women in this study did not feel supported by their friends, family and partners about breastfeeding. Once their children were born many women who initiated breastfeeding but stopped shortly afterwards said they stopped because of pressure of family and friends. (2012: 28)

Although I focus more on examples of extended family who actively or passive aggressively discourage EN, there are also many examples of friends and extended family who are supportive in different ways.

Friends

Among my interlocutors, most mentioned problems with talking openly about EN with their friends, in part because friends often had difficult experiences with initiating or maintaining chest/breastfeeding. Michelle, a physician/researcher, said that some of her friends "hated nursing. It was a source of stress," so they would say to her, "I don't know why you're still doing this." Among more distant friends, for example, "mom friends in the neighborhood," Michelle said they had all "stopped early." Crystal, a white woman with whom I exchanged messages privately after a social media interaction, wrote that,

> I have a mom friend who has breastfed two children and weaned them in the timeframe that I've nursed just my daughter. Any time I've had minor issues she tells me that I need to wean mine.

Richa, who was thirty-nine at the time of our in-depth interview, is an Indian American woman working in public health; she also did not have close friends who nursed for as long as she did with her two children. She said

> My peer group . . . a lot of them really had trouble . . . [I had] a lot of friends who said it didn't work for them. That was a little hard because I didn't have many friends who at that time [were also practicing EN].

Richa had weaned both of her children at the time of our interview, but she told me:

> I have a friend who said, "If I knew you then [when you were breastfeeding], I would have been judging you. Which is fine, we can joke about that sort of thing. And I say maybe I would be judging you too—she went like 6-9 months. But that's the joke we have between us—that if we'd known each other when our babies were first born, we would have totally judged each other.

Richa's comment demonstrates the fraught nature of talking openly about chest/breastfeeding with friends, since chest/breastfeeding initiation is very difficult for many people in the United States, as is maintaining the nursing relationship for more than a few weeks or months. Being aware of the struggles that other people might have had, I also rarely shared information with friends about my experiences when I was nursing.

Parents who practice EN sometimes find or make friends in in-person or online support groups, where people were able to talk or write openly about shared experiences. Stephanie mentioned that she followed a Facebook page ("The Badass Breastfeeder") and through that page, she found local spin-off groups that were very helpful. In private EN support groups, I saw numerous posts of people looking for "friends," as people would post that they did not have anyone in their friend group IRL (in real life) who understood the experience of EN and many who judged them if they talked about it. On some posts, I saw that people asked others to feel free to send friend requests so that they could expand their circle of supportive friends.

Extended Family

Extended family may feel more invested than friends or strangers in the long-term well-being of the child. They may be less likely to filter their opinions and may feel that their own plans related to the child or children will be affected by the parents'/direct caregivers' decisions. For many of my interlocutors, comments from extended family members about their decisions related to nursing often began when their children were still infants and ramped up over time. I start this section by recounting one of the more dramatic examples of a family member's attitudes about chest/breastfeeding in general, EN, and child-led weaning, and how they were expressed. One of my in-depth interviewees, Amy, PM'd me after seeing a comment I made on a chest/breastfeeding-friendly social media page, and we scheduled a time for a formal virtual interview about her EN experiences with her two children. Amy's story illustrates that this pressure can begin from day one and can indicate the degree to which popular beliefs and personal histories can leak into family relationships.

Amy, who self-identified as white and was forty-one at the time of our interview, worked full time as an attorney in the Midwest. She practiced EN with two children, and her three-year-old son had not yet weaned at the time of our interview. Despite several challenges she faced with her first child (a daughter), including a difficult labor and delivery and the discovery of an allergy in her younger child that prompted Amy to change her own diet, she continued to nurse her first child until she self-weaned. She told me that the hardest part of nursing did not have to do with these challenges but with her mother-in-law's attitude toward nursing and EN, with comments that came with the regularity of what Amy called a "negativity cuckoo clock." This was an interesting metaphor that captures both the relentless and repetitive nature of her mother-in-law's comments and the idea that the clock is ticking for a perceived "appropriate" duration of weaning, which fits into the neoliberal imaginary that children need to wean to be able to start the journey toward independence and self-actualization, with the accompanying beliefs by family that prolonged nursing holds the child (and the parent) back from eventually becoming a productive citizen.

Amy's mother-in-law (also white) came to stay with them for a short period after her first baby was born, and she frequently tried to insist on giving the baby a bottle or a pacifier, but Amy resisted this. After the first few weeks, Amy's mother-in-law started to suggest, "You might not make enough milk because you're small [in stature]." Amy would argue with her mother-in-law that her height was fairly average for women globally, and that "small" women had been able to nurse their children throughout history and prehistory. Then a barrage of comments would come at her, all of which reflected explanatory models about breastfeeding coupled with her mother-in-law's additional creative spins on these beliefs:

"You have small breasts, so you can't possibly make enough milk."
"Since you're nursing on-demand, you must be making skim milk."
"Because you ran during pregnancy, you might have a problem with your milk being shook up. You probably shook up the baby [in utero] running too."
"Because you're a vegetarian, you can't produce milk."
"You can't eat spicy foods and nurse."
"Because you never put her down, she can't nurse properly. You need to let her cry it out so you can have let down of your own milk."

When Amy's first baby was around ten weeks old, Amy did have some concerns about her daughter's weight but suspected it might be from her own consumption of dairy, since her (the baby's) cousin had tested positive for cow milk intolerance. She was encouraged to pump to see if it was more of a problem with her supply, but she insisted on a test, while agreeing to supplement with formula and pump. Her husband mentioned the test to his mother, and her "face lit up," and she said, "She's gonna bottle-feed!" It turned out her baby did test positive for this intolerance, but rather than switch to formula, Amy changed her diet and cut dairy, and things were fine after that.

Amy felt like she had to address each question and assertion that her mother-in-law introduced, so she frequently called a lactation hotline for information, to the point where they would answer, "What did your mother-in-law tell you this time?" She also attended LLL meetings and later became a certified La Leche leader. As her first child got older, Amy's saga continued with her mother-in-law often asking, unprompted: "Have you stopped torturing yourself yet?" Amy would say that she never once complained to anyone about her nursing experience. When she did have one issue with a clogged duct, she did not tell her mother-in-law as she knew it would be "I told you so." She and her husband started to set a strict schedule for visiting her mother-in-law—she would nurse in the car before visiting, and end the visit exactly after three hours. After just one year of nursing her first child, her mother-in-law said that now she had "met the deadline," she should be able to stop. One year was the recommended duration for chest/breastfeeding by the AAP at that time, but Amy told her mother-in-law that that was just a minimum they were recommending and not an upper limit.

As Amy continued to nurse, her mother-in-law would say, "You're making other people uncomfortable," when in reality, Amy did not share with anyone outside of the family that she was nursing. At one point, Amy had a work opportunity come up in which her in-laws accompanied her while they traveled, and Amy recalls her mother-in-law giving more reasons to wean while on this trip. Her mother-in-law was concerned continued nursing would make her daughter "clingy." Later, with her second child, Amy had the baby tested for cow milk intolerance early on. Her mother-in-law could not understand why she would "put herself through" a major dietary change when formula was available. Every time there was a gathering it got worse. Her mother-in-law would complain that night nursing created "babysitting issues" and would result in cavities.[2]

I asked Amy if she knew why her mother-in-law seemed so persistent in her anti-chest/breastfeeding agenda. She said that her husband's great-grandmother breastfed his grandmother up to age three—his grandmother had memories of herself (as a toddler) pulling up a chair to nurse from her mom. However, his grandmother bottle-fed his mother (Amy's mother-in-law). Amy said, "I'm not sure what changed," and we discussed some of the changes in infant feeding on a societal level when his mother was young, a time when formula was ubiquitous. With Amy's husband, her mother-in-law breastfed him as an infant exactly five times a day, a type of scheduled feeding that may have been recommended at the time (in the 1970s) but may be less than most babies need (both for their own nutrition and for the lactating parent to maintain a milk supply). After a few weeks, her mother-in-law said her own milk had "magically changed to water" and that it had "turned bad." Amy speculated that probably because she was not nursing on demand, her supply was low, and at a certain point, she had to switch to formula.

Despite the stated goal of wanting things to be easier for her daughter-in-law, Amy's mother-in-law introduced an excessive amount of emotional and intellectual labor for Amy to take on, especially during the first few years of her younger child's life; she had to constantly engage in the labor of justifying her choices. Amy had access to networks and knew how to access knowledge she could use to dispute the misinformation being given in the guise of caring, and Amy eventually sought additional education and training related to chest/breastfeeding and lactation.

Ashley, a white graduate student with three children who was originally from a lower-middle-class background, told me, in an in-depth interview we did in her home, about how her extended family had negative opinions about her nursing openly and about EN. Ashley was confident in her decisions to nurse her children and practice gentle weaning, but she said that her stepbrother and stepsister would often ask: "Well, how long are you gonna breastfeed? I'd be like, 'Well, when they're done.'" Ashley's stepmom also explicitly said that she should not nurse one of her sons at a family gathering when he was just a year old.

Ashley told me, "She [her stepmom] said, 'You know you *can't* nurse like that at my parents' party. You just can't.' And I was like, 'Well, I was gonna wear [a nursing-friendly] dress,' And she said, 'You just can't.' And it really bothered me. She was expecting me to hide somewhere." Ashley continued:

> So I wrote them this email saying that I was so sorry and I hope they wouldn't be offended but I wouldn't be attending . . . It came down to, "you think that it will offend people to breastfeed my child which is completely biological normal?"—and no one talked about it, but I felt weird toward my stepmom after that. Guess they're like super—the whitest people—all British and you know the kind of people with white napkins in their laps. So I ended up not going, and it might have ruffled some feathers but I just put it in an e-mail. And she just wrote back this response, "Oh, I'm so sorry we won't see you there."

Ashley's story parallels that of Amy and other people in online spaces who frequently write about simply avoiding family gatherings or contact in order to avoid the conflict or judgment from others related to their decision to nurse or practice child-led weaning. She also suggests that her stepmom's background, as British and maybe upper class/posh (signaled by the phrase "people with white napkins in their laps"), plays a part in her attitudes about nursing.

Family backgrounds, particularly for people with relatives from other countries, were mentioned by other interlocutors in terms of different impacts of stigma associated with EN. Although many countries have higher rates of exclusive breastfeeding for the first six months and longer average durations, this does not guarantee that there will be less stigma associated with EN for everyone, since the formula industry changed nursing practices globally in the twentieth century. The context of migration to the United States may also impact how stigma is felt and enacted in family contexts.

Richa and her husband are both Indian American, and their parents grew up in India. She found it surprising that her mother-in-law was uncomfortable with her nursing in front of her at home:

> The funny thing is, I didn't have a problem doing it in front of my mother-in-law, but she did. She thought I needed to be somewhere private. Like when we visited them, she would stand outside the door and talk to me if she needed something or she'd stand [turns away]. I was like, "really?". . . [I thought she] would have nursed more. I don't know what she did with her first two, because they were born in India and were there until they were like ten, twelve years old, but [Richa's husband] was born here—I don't know. She tells me that he was

given cereal in the hospital in his formula . . . He was a week old. How could that have been possible? . . . I think for all Indians, the privacy part of it, even though they may do it for a long time, the privacy aspect is big.

According to Mehta et al. (2017), extended nursing (also defined as beyond two years in their study) is common in India, but there has been a steady decrease in nursing duration over the past few decades. Social class plays a part in nursing practices as well; specifically, their study shows that both low-income and high-income women were more likely than middle-income women to nurse for more than two years, which they suggest may be related to the latter group being more likely to be working outside the home. There are complexities to every family's experience in terms of what they see as normal or abnormal, and immigration is another factor that can change how people understand and view infant and child feeding practices. Also, as Richa noted, privacy (and covering up) was more of an issue for her mother-in-law than nursing itself was. Horwood, et al. (2020), in a recent study of attitudes about breastfeeding among Indian families living and working in South Africa, found that women felt discouraged from nursing in public primarily because of local taboos associated with this practice, so it is possible that Richa's mother-in-law's experience with US taboos associated with nursing openly versus covering up was influenced by her time here.

Unlike Richa, Gabby, whose father is Black/African American and mother is Mexican American, found that her mother's family's cultural background/ethnicity played a positive role in her feeling comfortable in her nursing journey and with EN. Gabby, who was twenty-eight at the time of our virtual interview, was nursing her almost three-year-old and working full time as a medical assistant. She talked about feeling very supported by her mother and her mother's side of the family especially. She said she would hear stories from her Mexican family "like, 'oh, I breastfed for six years,'" so EN was never posited as strange or unusual. Her husband is white/of European descent, and she said that sometimes his family would make a comment like:

"Maybe you should stop, because she's older now." And then my side of the family was like, "No, keep going, she's doing great." It was not like a debate—it's like, everyone's supportive, but some people, like, have more ideas about it.

Harley et al. (2007), in a study of women "of Mexican descent" in the United States and nursing duration, found that the increase in the number of years of residence in the United States was correlated to a decrease in the duration of nursing, "including shorter duration of exclusive breastfeeding and any breastfeeding," with the lowest rates of nursing initiation and duration among those who were born in the United States. Gabby was born in the United States, but other circumstances (possibly her work in healthcare and support from her family and partner) may have contributed to her being able to and wanting to practice EN.

Jocelyn, a Filipina-American woman with whom I corresponded via PM after some posts she made in online support groups, grew up in the Philippines and practiced EN with her son. She said that in the Philippines,

> views on EN are also controversial. My mom who is a retired nurse thinks I should stop. My sister, an MD, used to tell me to stop until a retired medical child psychologist—her friend from med school—backed me up and said it is beneficial for my son to continue doing so.

As will be discussed in the next chapter, medical professionals often retain biases about EN with which they grew up.

Paige also experienced this issue with family members in the medical field:

> The most push back I've received is from my aunt, who is a registered nurse at [a university hospital]. She's adamant that breastfeeding is not beneficial after six months [and says that] they no longer get nutrients needed and that formula would support best after six months especially with babies' transition to solid foods. She doesn't have a background in Pediatrics. She is a cancer nurse. I have quoted the [AAP] and have discussed with her that my doctor agrees that it's best health wise if I can continue on as long as possible if it's good with me and baby.

Paige first told me (via PM) about her challenges with family members and later did a formal interview with me; her extended family had many opinions about her nursing her second child longer than what was considered "normal" in her family. Paige (white) grew up in a rural area of a Southeastern state. She believed that her relatives were mostly appalled by her "openness with it. [My son] refuses to be covered up and I really haven't ever put in any effort to hide feeding him." She said that most of the negative attention she received came from aunts, parents, grandparents, in-laws, and cousins:

> They were very supportive in the beginning—I was even praised for breastfeeding him. But around six months, I began to get questioned about when I was going to begin [weaning]. When I told them I wasn't [going to actively wean], I got a lot

of negative responses. At every family event, there is a huge conversation about it—I'm often confronted by several family members at once usually while I am openly feeding [my son]. They say the most absolutely ridiculous things, which doesn't last very long because I'm pretty strict on my stance. I also tend to answer with ridiculously sarcastic responses which tends to kill the conversation. Or my husband will step in to pull them away from me so I can breastfeed in peace.

Notably, having her partner (husband's) support, to be discussed in the next section, was significant in her being able to deal with these stigmatizing comments.

About a year after Paige and I first exchanged messages about her family pressuring her to wean, she messaged me about new ways her family had found to disparage her decision to practice EN with her son. He had received an autism diagnosis and was nonverbal, and family members tried to blame EN. They would say:

"Do you think you breast feeding him so long is why he doesn't talk? Because he spent so much time nursing instead of talking." Or "I wonder if there is any correlation between autism and breastfeeding. Bet they won't publish that data!" Or "I bet he has autism because you got that Covid vaccine while you were pregnant but honestly he seemed normal until you got your Covid booster. I wonder if the booster caused the autism because you were breastfeeding him. Did they say you could breastfeed and get the Covid booster?"

Paige's ability to defend and feel comfortable with her decision to continue nursing her son was bolstered by her education. She had her first child when she was still in high school but managed to complete her degree and go straight to college (as a first-generation college student) and later graduate school to get a Master's and find a job in her field in her early twenties. As with most of my in-depth interviewees, the cultural and social capital she acquired during this process made it possible (if not easy) for her to stand up to relatives and to be less likely to internalize the messages that they were doing something that could harm their child.

Jenny, a white dental health professional who posted in an EN online support group and with whom I was in touch through PM, expressed her extreme frustration with her mother-in-law, who cared for her child during the day. Her mother-in-law often put pressure on her to wean her child. Her child had a cavity, and the mother-in-law blamed Jenny, who was practicing EN and night nursing. As someone working in the dental field, Jenny felt strongly that the reason for the cavity was not because of night nursing but because her mother-in-law frequently gave her child processed foods and sweet drinks, despite Jenny's urging that only water should be given. From Jenny's perspective, her mother-in-law ignored and undermined Jenny's own professional expertise and knowledge and, from Jenny's perspective, was sabotaging her child's dental health, but Jenny said she could not afford to pay for alternative childcare. The role that grandparents and other members of the extended family sometimes play in childcare can have a significant impact on parents who practice EN. The financial benefits of having this type of assistance can come with the cost of losing some agency in decision-making related to feeding and other parenting decisions.

Relatives who do not live close by or who cannot play a significant role in daily childcare may also want to have children stay at their homes or vacation with them. Since overnights away from the nursing parent can be difficult for children, particularly if they are used to night nursing or at least falling asleep to nurse, relatives might pressure EN parents to wean before their children are ready. My own parents were very supportive of nursing, but they also wanted my son to be able to sleep over at their house or at their hotel when they came to visit, and his not being able to fall asleep without milk sometimes made this more complicated. We were able to work this out as my son got older and did not often wake up at night once he fell asleep; a few times I would nurse him to sleep at their hotel and then leave, and they were very supportive of this solution.

Kim, a 46-year-old white woman with a degree in engineering, gave an example of how her parents were similarly supportive of her EN journey. She said that when she was in the process of trying to gently wean her three-and-a-half-year-old, her parents wanted to make sure that her choice to wean was not coming from pressure:

> And my mom even had read some kind of article about how much longer like, that basically is natural up to, like, age seven or something. You know, and she was like, "hey, just, you know, [so] you don't feel like we've been encouraging you to [wean]."

Kim said her mom had chest/breastfed her and her siblings but had taken a more active role in weaning her own children, but she only shared the story of this when asked by Kim. Her mom stopped nursing Kim and one of her siblings because of pregnancy with the next child and, with her youngest, when he was almost three, she sent him with their dad and siblings to the beach for a week, and when he came back, he had lost interest in her milk. Kim's mom wanted her to know, however, that she and Kim's father were supportive of her decision to practice child-led weaning.

EN parents who are open about their nursing experiences on their social media pages often experience pushback from family members. Cyberbullying related to nursing and EN is common in public forums online, but many of the most harmful and hateful comments seem to take place on personal social media accounts. In private support groups, it is common for people practicing EN to include a statement like, "I can't post this on my personal page because my family wants me to wean" or "my family thinks that what I'm doing is wrong." Members of these groups will give examples of friends and relatives blocking them or unfriending them after they posted a photo or a comment about chest/breastfeeding their toddler or child, including sharing milestones of how long they have been nursing (which are very much celebrated by others in private support groups). I have seen posts also that encourage fellow members to share on personal pages, in an effort to further normalize the practice and help others who may have questions about EN or child-led weaning, but this level of openness can lead to backlash and can affect relationships.

Allison, a white mom of two, posted in an EN support group about negative comments she received after posting on her personal page about nursing her two-year-old son. She noted that a few people among her Facebook friends (including family members) would always post comments about the need for her to wean so that he would be able to "develop" normally. She said that it was frustrating and disheartening because she had made a choice to post on her personal page to help normalize the practice but got constant criticism. She said she was not embarrassed about EN, but she felt bad that people she was close to would repeatedly make critical comments anytime she posted about it.

In online spaces, I noticed that hostile sexism, as discussed in Chapter 2, is common in some of the language that people use when making a comment about it was time to wean. Often (but not exclusively) these comments came from cisgender men who are also friends or family members, and they would often use more vulgar and colloquial terms in relation to breasts or the act of nursing when they felt that this nursing relationship should come to an end. They might say it was time to "get off the tit" or time to "stop sucking your mommy's tit." These are colloquial phrases commonly used in the United States to signify the need for someone to stop being dependent on others or the government and fit into the wider cultural imaginary that suggests that weaning represents an independence that must be achieved for a child to self-actualize. The use of the term "tit" for breast is often used by men in a sexual or degrading way. Another common comment in online spaces is that if a child is old enough to know the "true purpose of breasts" (implying for a partner's sexual satisfaction), they should be weaned. More often, these types of comments are directed at feminine-presenting individuals who are chest/breastfeeding boys or children assigned male at birth.

Although overtly sexist comments like this may be more common online, there are also family members who are comfortable making these comments in person, in front of a child who is nursing and sometimes directly to the child, perhaps as an example of a more "benevolent sexism" (Glick and Fiske 1996), a sort of paternalistic stance that protects women from the child (or alternatively, this could be interpreted as more "hostile" in its intent to protect the child from the woman/parent). Paige mentioned that both her father and her father-in-law would make these types of negative comments:

> The men [in my family] have made comments like, oh, "he's just gonna be a titty man. He's looking for titties, and I'm like, I think that's a sensory thing—like that feeling of squishing—it was almost like a stress ball, you know. That's a familiar, comforting thing that he may recognize from breastfeeding, and that's why he's drawn to it, but I don't think it's him trying to, like, you know, cop a feel or something. It's not. Yeah, it's I think it's absolutely a comfort thing.

Paige saw her son's squeezing or "squishing" her breasts while nursing as providing a specific form of comfort for him because he is autistic; however, "twiddling" the nipple of the other breast and seeming to "play with" or squeeze the lactating parent's breast while nursing is very common, since young children as they "develop their fine motor skills, calm themselves and occupy themselves . . . Some stroke, some pull, some rub between a finger and thumb" (Pickett 2024: 41). When viewed by people who have never been exposed to what this looks like (and for whom women's breasts are seen as primarily sexual objects), it is unsurprising that they interpret a boy grabbing or squeezing his mother's breast as related to sexual desire.

Partners/Spouses

Support of a partner/partners is important to breastfeeding and is very helpful to the EN relationship. Les'Shon Irby's research focused on the importance of the support of fathers in a small but diverse sample of families in the state of Georgia (United States). Cisgender fathers (non-lactating parents) did not play a large role in making the decision that their wives/partners would nurse their children, but postpartum support by fathers assisted in the continuation of nursing (Irby 2016;Irby et al. 2019). In my sample from in-depth interviews of people practicing EN, spousal or partner support was present for breastfeeding and EN among most participants with the exception of one woman for whom custody issues threatened the nursing relationship with her youngest child, which I will discuss in more depth in Chapter 6 on legal issues. The rest had general support for their nursing journey from their partners; from the narratives that emerged from interviews, it was clear that every one of my in-depth interviewees expected this type of support from partners and were also the primary decision-makers in relation to breastfeeding and weaning decisions. However, this does not mean there were never any issues related to EN in these relationships.

My own experience and Irby's research led me to pay attention to the many comments online about spousal and partner support or lack thereof. Even in supportive relationships, EN parents talked/wrote about struggles and doubts their non-lactating partners would have at one point or another. Anne, a white woman, was thirty-nine at the time of our in-depth interview and was working full time as a nurse. Her older child had weaned, but she was still nursing her three-year-old. She noted that her husband was extremely supportive of her nursing both of her children, but at the same time, she said, "I don't think he expected it to go on quite this long" or to be as complicated as it was, particularly with co-sleeping. A common theme among both interviewees and people in online support groups is that after a few years, their partner was ready for them to "be done." Because of the intimate nature of the partner relationship, there is usually a different dynamic with partners than with extended family. This intimacy may include daily proximity, sexual and romantic intimacy, and sharing of physical spaces, especially related to sleeping. In my own relationship, my husband was generally supportive of nursing and EN for me in theory. Also an anthropologist, he did not think of co-sleeping or child-led weaning as abnormal or disgusting. At the same time, he sometimes complained of how both of these parenting practices created disruptions to our sleep patterns and ability to have date nights.

Support from spouses can include both the theoretical support for EN and child-led weaning and a willingness to attempt to empathize and learn about the complicated nature of these practices and to make an effort to assist with caregiving practices when possible. Some EN parents talked or wrote about how partners thought that chest/breastfeeding made it hard for them to play a role in childcare and bedtime routines during the early years of their child's life, though there are many ways these roles can be shared. Melissa had two children from her first husband and two from her current husband, and she practiced EN with all of her children. Both of her partners, she said, were supportive of her decisions to practice EN and child-led weaning, though with both, she said,

> There's always the moment where you have to explain to your husband how important the milk is . . . there's always that moment where they leave a bottle [of pumped milk] out [of the fridge, which could make it unusable] and they don't understand exactly why you're so upset about it and you have to explain it to them. Yeah. It's like golden.

Her current husband also helped support tandem nursing of her two youngest children by playing an important role in sharing caregiving roles at night:

> My husband would have the little baby, and I would have [my older son] in the back, and I would nurse him to sleep. And then I would send a text to my husband, and my husband put the little baby down and come get [the older child] from me and put him in the bed so that he wouldn't wake up. But, like, it took him forever to fall asleep.

This kind of partnership takes at least some of the burden off the lactating parent and allows the non-lactating parent to bond with their children.

Michelle said that her husband, like her, was a research scientist and was aware of the health benefits of nursing their child, though she said that this, "completely let him off the hook for everything for the first three months," referring to the fact that she had the primary responsibility of waking up with their infant to nurse. However, he did not want the baby in the bed with them, so after having her son in a bassinet in the same room for a while, they moved him to a different room upstairs where she would nurse him to sleep and eventually she could put him to sleep in a crib. She also said:

> I wonder if my husband thinks that, you know, maybe nursing him for so long I like prolonged his babyhood and that that's why he's so—he's like a little barnacle, a clingy barnacle still.

Kim's husband also "kind of made a big push for us to be done when [their daughter] was around two," but Kim felt that she was nursing so much at that point that she was not ready. She told him to stop telling their daughter that she would have to stop nursing soon. Her husband accepted that—or rather, "he gave up on intervening" in terms of saying anything directly to their child about it.

The lack of serious complaints about spousal support among my in-depth interviews may be a result of a skewed sample of interview participants in the study who were well-informed and who would not accept a partner who did not accept their parenting choices. However, on social media private support groups for EN, comments about lack of spousal or partner support appear almost daily. This may be a skewed sample as well, since support groups are places where people generally come to seek help, whereas they might not come to the group with the intention of posting examples of everything that is going well. Concerns and complaints from partners fall generally into a few categories: concerns for the child's well-being (physical, emotional, or developmental); concerns that are more about the partner (e.g., limitations that EN presents in terms of sexual activity, time, travel, and affection or sleeping/comfort issues); and embarrassment or shame, often stemming from things their own friends or relatives say to them. There is sometimes a concern among partners that EN will also forever alter the shape and appearance of a lactating person's breasts. In online support groups, I saw several stories of more violent actions from partners, including physical abuse and abusive language related to EN. Verbal abuse, including the use of sexist language as discussed above, is commonly mentioned by participants in these spaces, and I have seen a few examples of people posting in support groups about incidents in which their child was physically ripped away from their breast by a partner.

I also asked interviewees and read comments online about sexual intimacy issues. Non-lactating partners sometimes had aversions to sexual intimacy because their partner was chest/breastfeeding, even if they were otherwise supportive. In the United States in particular, we learn from an early age that feminine breasts are an object of sexual arousal and interest, and there is a cognitive adjustment that is necessary for someone to come to see breasts as the vehicle for feeding a child and not (or at least not solely) for sexual pleasure. In online spaces and other pages dedicated to breastfeeding, a common trope is the assertion that breasts are body parts whose primary function is to feed children and that they are "not sexual"; others, however, have mentioned breasts as playing a part in their own adult sex lives, but sometimes after nursing a child for several years, they are less comfortable with a partner engaging with breasts during sex. Among my in-depth interviewees, however, the discomfort was more often coming from partners. Deanna mentioned that her partner did change the way he interacted with her in terms of sexual intimacy when she was nursing her son, and she said that "it was pissing me off because I didn't feel like a different person, you know what I mean? But he got to a point where it was kind of like, 'well, those [breasts] are for him' [her son]."

Kim said that co-sleeping with her daughter (in a different bed from her husband) was the main reason that their sex life was affected:

> Probably, in the biggest way is that we're not reliably alone in our bed ever. You know, we typically will have like, a Friday night date night . . . you know, a couple times a month, we'll go out.

Kim also talked about the challenges of getting a child to sleep, which also often comes with frequent waking: "I'll work hard to get out of her room when she falls asleep because again, like, she will fall asleep with my boob in her mouth. And so there's an extraction process." She also mentioned changes related to EN or having children in general, such as early menopause and changes in sleep practices ("Before she was born, we slept naked, you know?") as intersecting factors that affected sexual intimacy with her husband.

The Labor of Standing up to Family and Friends

The primary theme that emerged from interviews and participant observation in online spaces is that, even for those who feel supported by family and friends, much of the intellectual labor in both acquiring knowledge and crafting ways to explain and justify not only EN but also chest/breastfeeding practices in general to other family members is performed by the lactating parent. Returning to Amy's story of her struggle with her mother-in-law's opinions, one might wonder about her husband's perspectives in the constant barrage of comments and urgings to wean from her mother-in-law/his mother. She said he was supportive for the most part, but just as Amy grew more confident in knowing what was working for her child, her mother-in-law's words started sowing seeds of doubt in her husband's mind. She said she "knew enough from La Leche meetings, but my husband didn't know." As their child thrived, she said that her husband stopped worrying and has been very supportive of her nursing journey. Notably, he did not himself do research on his own but was "convinced" after seeing that his child turned out fine. However, he was influenced by Amy's advocacy to the point where he later applied the information in his own workplace to advocate for accommodations for nursing parents.

A few of my participants in in-depth interviews sought professionalization skills and certifications in lactation or child nutrition or even changed their career paths after their experience with EN or otherwise sought knowledge they could share with others. The time and effort that are involved in data gathering for justifying one's decisions to friends and family members or in becoming a La Leche leader or getting an IBCLC certification are not available to everyone. Social class and access to social and cultural capital can contribute to whether someone is able to either demonstrate to family and friends that their parenting decisions related to EN and weaning are not harmful to their children or to be able to continue chest/breastfeeding with confidence in their decisions despite what family and friends think or say. Having support from some family members (especially a spouse or partner) can sometimes be enough to make it easier for someone to practice EN. In online spaces, I also saw many people mention that they "gave in" to family pressure at some point and weaned before they or their child were ready, but participants in online support groups also frequently reach out to collect information and seek validation to strengthen their resolve in their own decision-making when it comes to family members who disagree with their choices. Many people in these groups also spend a significant amount of time answering others' questions with extensive details and resources. The need for self-advocacy and significant intellectual labor to manage EN stigma was also apparent in the medical encounter, as will be demonstrated in the next chapter.

5

Encounters with Biomedicine

Support, Shame, Stigma, and Iatrogenic Harm

When we went for a third-year checkup for my son, the pediatrician on call said that I no longer needed to breastfeed. I said we were doing child-led weaning. She said, 'you know there are kids who are five and older who will just jerk down their mother's top to get milk, so you should wean before you find yourself in that situation.' She said that I need to stop now and switch to cow's milk and talked about it as if it would only take a few days of listening to him cry for milk, and he would be weaned.

The above quotation is paraphrased from a post (with consent from the woman, pseudonym Meg, a white woman from the Midwest who posted in an EN support group online). The description of her visit to the pediatrician mirrors many other incidents that lactating parents describe in the medical encounter. In this case, Meg was confident in her own decisions and had participated in EN support groups on Facebook since before her child turned one. In this post, rather than asking for advice and validation, she was expressing her frustration with this physician's rude way of discussing the issue, including the suggestion that "switching to cow's milk" was a necessary step for the child's health, and that abrupt weaning was the answer.

This frustration, frequently articulated by parents who practice EN, exemplifies the experience of discussing EN with some biomedical doctors and other healthcare professionals in the United States. Feelings of shame and guilt are induced or exacerbated for people practicing EN when a healthcare professional tells them that EN is not only weird or unnecessary but that it could potentially contribute to a physical or psychological problem. EN parents in online support groups describe interactions with healthcare professionals that reinforce their family or friends' opinions that "at this point, you're just doing it for yourself." In *Others' Milk: The Potential of Exceptional Breastfeeding*, sociologist Kristin Wilson noted that while parents are strongly encouraged by the biomedical community to nurse children during their infancy, the

> mutual construction of breastfeeding and institutional authority starts to leak when breastfeeders violate any of the spoken or unspoken social norms of institutional rules in order to breastfeed—in effect, when their breastfeeding becomes "exceptional" (2018: 6).

In addition to the intellectual and emotional labor that often goes into standing up to family members who might be unsupportive of EN decisions, people who are chest/breastfeeding in non-normative ways "do intense moral work at the boundaries of what society deems acceptable" (Wilson 2018: 6) in their interactions with pediatricians, dentists, and other healthcare professionals.

Some healthcare professionals' responses about EN have to do with the shock they encounter upon finding out that a child is still chest/breastfeeding beyond what they expect is "normal." Interview participants and people in EN support groups online described instances of healthcare professionals reacting in negative ways to the fact that they were still nursing, often well before the two-year mark that I used to define EN for this project. Many EN parents do try to counter healthcare professionals' statements about nursing with information they have gathered from their own research or experiences. Most commonly, they cite the WHO's recommendation that children receive breast milk for two years or more, to which it seems common for healthcare professionals to respond, "Ok, but that recommendation is for Africa" or "for the Third World" or "for the developing world, where children would die without it." Most of the data collected for this book took place before a more recent AAP's 2022 recommendation of nursing for two years or more, "as long as you and your baby desire" (Feldman-Winter 2024: Online).

Reported statements (told from the perspective of people practicing EN) that healthcare providers make often reflect common societal beliefs and lack of exposure to the practice of EN. There is often a notable difference between the explanatory models that many biomedical professionals in the United States have about EN and the information that is available through national and international health organizations. The latter tend to be more in line with both the lived experience of people who practice EN and healthcare professionals who specialize in lactation and child nutrition. I use the term "biomedicine" here in a way that is typically used by medical anthropologists to describe a system of medicine that originated in the Western context that emphasizes a science-based approach to understanding the body, health, and disease (Gaynes and Davis-Floyd

2004). "Biomedicine" suggests the fact that this form of medicine is practiced globally (not just in the "West"), though "Western medicine" is often still used as a synonym in some contexts. "Allopathic medicine" and "cosmopolitan medicine" are other terms in use as synonyms for biomedicine. Medical anthropologists also acknowledge that although biomedicine is based on scientific, evidence-based research, it can be as flawed and biased as those who practice it and the historical and political context in which it is practiced. The interpretation of scientifically collected data that informs both policy and biomedical practice can also be flawed and biased, though it is possible to identify the historical and contemporary sources of some aspects of bias. In this chapter, I start by discussing some of the potential negative impacts or "iatrogenic harm" that can result from both knowledge gaps and biases that exist among many healthcare professionals related to EN, followed by examples of iatrogenic harm as told primarily from the perspectives of my interlocutors. I describe some of the ways EN parents manage stigma in the biomedical encounter, and I include some examples of healthcare professionals who take a more collaborative approach with EN parents.

Iatrogenic Harm and Other Stressful Encounters with Biomedicine

"Iatros" is the Greek word for "physician," but "iatrogenic" is often used more broadly to apply to something that comes out of the broader interaction with the biomedical system. Philosopher Ivan Illich, in his book *Medical Nemesis* (1974) and many other publications, used the term "iatrogenesis" to refer to harm that is brought about by medical practices and procedures. Illich suggested that iatrogenesis also might emerge from medical policy. In subsequent discussions of this concept by medical anthropologists, "iatrogenic" is often used as an adjective in conjunction with "harm," "violence," or "stigma." Norman Sartorius (2002) wrote a seminal paper on "iatrogenic stigma" as it applies to the psychiatric profession; he pointed out how both the language that is often used in psychiatry to refer to mental illness and the extreme side effects of commonly prescribed medications further contribute to associated stigma and harm. Sartorius' work had an impact on my thoughts on Hansen's disease/leprosy stigma, which often is not simply about societal stigma associated with the disease itself but also about the many ways that the medical encounter and the medical community exacerbate or create new forms of stigma (White 2008).

In assessing "harm" in this chapter, I am focusing primarily on the perceptions of the lactating caregivers who are the target population of this study. Harm can take the form of emotional or psychological stress, physical harm, or the risk of both. For example, participants in this study considered abrupt weaning, particularly for toddlers and older children, to be a potentially traumatic event both for them and for their children, and some had had a negative experience with abrupt weaning of at least one child. For them, the mandate to wean abruptly (as opposed to child-led or gentle weaning practices) was seen as not only an attempt to strip them of their autonomy but also as harmful to their child and to them. Other forms of potential iatrogenic harm can arise from clinicians telling caregivers they must wait to take a medication, get surgery, or have a diagnostic test until they have weaned, when there is no evidence-based justification for them to either wait or wean before their child is ready.

In the larger online support groups for people who practice EN, there are daily posts by members of the groups about healthcare professionals telling them they should stop chest/breastfeeding, often "as soon as possible." The reasoning can vary—from general concerns about the physical and/or psychological/emotional health of the child or lactating parent to specific concerns related to a medication or medical procedure. Based on an analysis of thousands of posts, it is clear that there are biomedical professionals in the United States who do not attempt to access peer-reviewed studies or recommendations by the WHO or the AAP but instead draw directly on assumptions based on popular models of EN. Others might draw on knowledge or information they might have acquired in medical school that is now considered outdated or incomplete. There is still a notable discrepancy between the information that biomedical professionals are telling nursing parents in the United States and the most recent, evidence-based data on chest/breastfeeding and weaning; this discrepancy can be at least partially understood as deriving from a set of morals and preconceived ideas that posits EN as unnecessary and that reflect a lack of exposure to EN among healthcare professionals (both in their own experience and that of their patients).

Biomedical healthcare professionals often bring some of the ideas they learned as they were growing up to their practice. This is especially true for health-related conditions that are less commonly discussed in medical school or for which there is still a degree of ambiguity in the published literature. Within "critical medical anthropology," in which biomedicine is acknowledged to be influenced by different historical, political, social, and economic forces, medical anthropologists often document the ways that healthcare professionals' explanatory models of health, illness, and the body are shaped at least in part by unconscious biases and popular beliefs. Through participant observation that took place as part of her work as a communicable disease investigator for the county health department in a Southwestern state of the United States, medical anthropologist Susan McCombie found that "flu" typically meant something different to laypeople versus epidemiologists, but that laypeople's understanding was not unlike that of physicians. For laypeople, "the flu" was a "ready label that can be applied to almost any kind of febrile illness" (1987: 989), and she noticed that doctors use a similar label ("viral syndrome"), which corresponds to the folk model of "flu" and is used as a diagnostic label, typically in the absence of a definitive diagnosis. She noted that "[p]hysicians use explanatory models in actual practice that are divergent from scientific explanatory models and closely related to popular models of illness" (1987: 982).

In research I conducted in Brazil and the United States on Hansen's disease (leprosy), I found that healthcare professionals who had specialized in Hansen's disease were knowledgeable about diagnostic signs of the disease and its treatment. However, people affected by the disease described interactions with non-specialist healthcare professionals who had little knowledge of Hansen's disease beyond popular beliefs (for example, that it is highly contagious, that a person diagnosed with the disease should be isolated from others, and that there is no cure). Expectations by physicians that a person with Hansen's disease would "look" a certain way—as portrayed in popular media, in the Bible, in film and television, which typically represent advanced, untreated cases of the disease—generate iatrogenic harm as people are often misdiagnosed with allergies, rheumatoid arthritis, lupus, or other diseases because early signs of Hansen's disease do not match with the popular explanatory model (White 2009).

Stereotypes that are part of wider cultural imaginaries about racial identity also inform attitudes of biomedical professionals toward patients. For example, the idea among some healthcare professionals that African Americans have a higher pain tolerance because they have "thicker skin" or have come to be more physiologically resilient (which is also a popular belief about racial differences) can result in under-prescribing of pain medication and inattentiveness to the needs of Black patients in hospitals in the United States (Hoffman et al. 2016). Dána-Ain Davis documented birth stories about Black women in the United States that demonstrate that these beliefs that healthcare professionals hold, in addition to causing overt discrimination and microaggressions in medical settings, form the many "[l]ayers of obstetric racism" (Davis 2019: 567) that contribute to higher rates of maternal mortality for Black women than any other group in the United States.

In their recent book, *Lazy, Crazy, and Disgusting: Stigma and the Undoing of Global Health*, Alexandra Brewis and Amber Wutich discuss how popular perceptions and societal expectations about a variety of health-related conditions also impact biomedical care. In discussing "obesity" and "overweight" as concepts, for example, they note that stigma associated with fatness has increased in recent years, and this stigma is commonly reinforced in medical school training. This in turn impacts how healthcare professionals interact with patients:

> Given the cultural myth that obesity is always extremely unhealthy, clinicians often focus on an obese patient's weight during consultations even if the patient is there for entirely unrelated reasons. Similarly, slimmer people with unhealthy metabolic profiles are often not counseled to make lifestyle changes, because their doctors assume they are healthy. As one of our bariatric study participants put it, "You know, you go in there, 'I got a headache.' [The doctor says] 'It's because you're fat.' 'My toes hurt.' 'It's because you're fat.'" The website First Do No Harm is replete with people's stories of doctors refusing to diagnose and treat serious illnesses because they remain convinced that any health problem in someone classified as obese must stem from their weight. Take Katie, for example, whose walking pneumonia was missed because the doctor was convinced she had obesity-triggered sleep apnea. Or Rachel, who was congratulated for losing so much weight, which turned out to be the result of debilitating Crohn's disease. Or Erica, who was struck by a drunk driver and seriously injured, but the ER doctor decided he couldn't set her broken arm because of her size. (2019: 103)

It is noteworthy that the examples given here are all of women or people with feminine names, as gender identity also plays a large part in how patients are treated or whether they are taken seriously in the biomedical encounter.

Medical anthropologist Leah Ashe (2021) detailed her own experience with iatrogenic harm in an autoethnographic account of her involuntary stay in a UK hospital. Ashe described how healthcare professionals made incorrect assumptions that she had an eating disorder and would not listen to her explanations of chronic intestinal problems that had led to weight loss; their assumptions, in part based on what they "expected" the problem to be, based on her profile as a young woman who experienced extreme weight loss, prompted a number of procedures that removed her agency and made her essentially a prisoner of the healthcare system (which may have contributed to her untimely death).

Gender-based assumptions by biomedical practitioners also have implications for people practicing EN, the majority of whom are feminine-presenting. While trans men and transmasculine people in the United States sometimes describe some degree of male privilege in certain arenas of daily life (Clements et al. 2022), they may also be feminized by clinicians because of their status as a birthing parent and/or lactating caregiver. Yet when AFAB men seek gender-affirming care, medical professionals make assumptions about whether that gender transition is about an essentialized set of gender roles; clinicians tend to revert to stereotypes of what are "essentially" masculine or feminine roles. In a study of trans and nonbinary people in Canada who went through pregnancy, many of whom also nursed their children, one respondent said:

> To get top surgery you kind of have to talk about it as if you never want to get pregnant, right, to the surgeon. You can't be wiggly about that so I don't know . . . I don't think there was a way to talk to him about getting surgery without having a conventional narrative about it. [Felix]. (in MacDonald et al. 2016: 5 of online article)

In other words, many medical professionals maintain beliefs about the gender binary—that those who give birth and nurse their children are by nature "women" or "feminine." MacDonald et al. described iatrogenic stigma and harm that is generated in many medical encounters with transfeminine people:

> Providers need to be aware that the act of breastfeeding or chestfeeding is not necessarily perceived as feminine by their transmasculine clients. From the interviews, we see a distinction between gender dysphoria rooted in the individual's feelings about their body versus gender dysphoria triggered by social interactions. This distinction has important implications for health care providers. It means that care providers and others are capable of causing gender dysphoria in patient by misgendering them. Conversely, care providers can affirm a patient's gender identity through appropriate language, respectful touch, and other intentional actions, and thus alleviate distress associated with gender dysphoria. (2016: 14 of online article)

They go on to discuss ways that providers can facilitate chest/breastfeeding for the short and long term for transmasculine individuals by being aware of the specific health issues that trans people might face during different stages in their transition.

For people practicing EN, navigating multiple sets of recommendations (from friends, family, healthcare professionals, and online sources) is especially challenging. The authoritative nature of the biomedical encounter can make it difficult for parents to question directives from healthcare professionals unless they feel confident in their own ability to do research on their own or access other social networks. Support groups online are especially helpful in terms of sharing information. EN parents, especially those who have nursed more than one child for many years, also draw on their lived experience to counter or critique healthcare professionals' advice or mandates to wean before the parent and child/children are ready. However, those who do not have access to these resources might go with doctors' orders without question, especially if they do not also have a supportive family or friend group.

In digital ethnographic analysis and in-depth interviews, people practicing EN often said that they did not discuss chest/breastfeeding with healthcare professionals unless it was necessary, but there are many circumstances in which they were asked or they felt compelled to reveal that they were still nursing. The following sections, organized according to forms of healthcare for children (pediatric general health and pediatric dentistry) and healthcare for the lactating parent (including discussions of certain conditions, prescriptions, and medical procedures), contain examples of circumstances that most typically prompted a discussion with healthcare professionals about the need to wean or about the need to wait on a procedure or treatment until their children were weaned. I focus on practitioners of US-based biomedicine. Healers or practitioners from other medical traditions might also push for early weaning under some circumstances, but the majority of posts that I have observed in support groups are about encounters with biomedicine. In online groups over the years, I found only one mention of an alternative/holistic medical practitioner (a holistic dentist who was encouraging night weaning for cavities). The frequency with which some themes appear on social media sites and in the narratives of my interlocutors for in-depth interviews demonstrates that the cultural imaginary of the "need to wean" for a child to be healthy and to mature is common within the biomedical community in the United States.

Child Wellness and Pediatrician Encounters

In the first several years of a child's life, parents and children in the United States typically have several encounters with pediatricians. Most doctors, including pediatricians, receive limited training in medical school to support chest/breastfeeding. According to Gary et al. (2017: 164), much of what a medical student learns about breastfeeding medicine is highly dependent on specific patient encounters and the expertise of attending physicians, rather than a formal breastfeeding education curriculum.

Pediatricians can also inadvertently contribute to early weaning through unnuanced warnings against co-sleeping, night nursing, and nursing a child to sleep. The pediatricians at the practice where I took my son encouraged chest/breastfeeding and never expressed negative sentiments about EN, but they discouraged me from nursing him to sleep (even while sitting up/in a rocking chair). One pediatrician told me to put him down in his crib just as he seemed to get sleepy but before he was completely asleep. In practice, this suggestion seemed absurd to me and did not work for my son as an infant, as he would immediately start crying and would then be fully awake or throwing up within a minute or two. We used a kind of "sidecar" bed initially, instead of the crib, and after my son got older, we moved our mattress to the floor and removed heavy blankets and pillows for safer co-sleeping/bedsharing.

Telling parents that they need to nurse "on a schedule" rather than "on demand" is another recommendation that can lead to early weaning. Asking parents to track how much and how many times a day a baby is drinking is a recommendation that does not work well for chest/breastfeeding parents who are nursing primarily from the body. With bottle feeding, it is possible to keep track of the exact amount an infant is consuming. For parents who are practicing exclusive nursing from the body, it is not possible to know the amount the child is getting through the breast. I remember being frustrated in attempting to track the number of times my son wanted to nurse, because especially in the first few months, this seemed to happen nonstop around the clock. I later learned these frequent and sustained nursing sessions are known as "cluster feeding," which typically happen during infant growth spurts. In a study in South Africa, Sebitosi-Van Jaarsveled (2022) focused on knowledge about cluster feeding among mothers and healthcare workers. She found that over half of the healthcare workers in her sample did not know the word "cluster feeding," and though some were aware of growth spurts, they did not always understand when these typically occur or how they related to feeding frequency. Cluster feeding, in my experience, made it more difficult to know how to "count" the number of feedings in a day—was it two, nearly continuous sessions that lasted four to six hours or twenty sessions with small breaks in between? Sometimes on social media support groups, parents would joke that in answer to how many times a day their child nursed, they would say something like, "I don't know. One million?" If parents or healthcare workers misinterpret frequent or prolonged nursing sessions as the child "not getting enough" milk, they may try to supplement with formula, which can in some cases lead to early weaning.

Several posts and comments have to do with certain metrics of growth (e.g., weight gain) that may be based on formula-fed babies. Pediatricians are often unaware of what is "typical" or "normal" for babies that receive human milk. Michelle, a physician herself, said she had no problems initiating nursing, despite her son being born via C-section, but he was slow to gain weight and was still very small at thirty-nine weeks. Instead of supplementing with formula, she was able to pump her own milk to increase her supply and do a mix of bottle feeding with nursing from the breast. In our interview, we discussed standards for infant weight, and she mentioned that the AAP uses "growth charts . . . that are not WHO—they're based on babies in Ohio in the fifties or something like that." This was mentioned in a *New York Times* article (Carroll 2020: Online) that noted that growth charts created in 1977 were based on a small sample of "white, middle-class infants living in southwest Ohio." In this article, the author does note that these charts were revised in 2000 to include a broader sample of children from the United States. The WHO produced new charts in 2006, "focusing on how kids should grow under optimal conditions (such as being breastfed and living in safe, comfortable, smoke-free homes)." The CDC in the United States "recommended in 2010 that pediatricians start using the WHO charts until children were 2, and then switch back to CDC charts after that" (Carroll 2020: Online). In general, Michelle's point speaks to the problematic nature of physicians' strict interpretations of growth charts as "facts" about what constitutes a normal range for growth since the normal range might change significantly based on the population sampled.

Pediatrician instructions, in this case based on AAP recommendations, for separate sleeping arrangements can also result in early weaning. This is a more complicated aspect of what pediatricians tell parents because the recommendations they learn and that they pass on to patients come from an authoritative source and are often presented as very cut and dry, or rather, a life-and-death message of absolutes. To prevent Sudden Infant Death Syndrome, parents are told to place infants on their backs "in their own sleep space," like "a crib, bassinet or portable play yard with a firm, flat mattress and a fitted sheet," with no "loose blankets, pillows, stuffed toys, bumpers and other soft items." While having a bassinet that attaches to the lactating parent's bed is not contraindicated, co-sleeping in general, and bed sharing in particular, is constructed as extremely dangerous because of the risks of adults accidentally smothering the infant through overlaying or smothering from blankets or pillows (AAP 2024: Online). Anthropologist James McKenna has argued that co-sleeping and chest/breastfeeding are more protective against infant death than sleeping separately, but certain variables are associated with increased risk, and "a consistent feature associated with populations where bedsharing and high infant deaths co-exist is extreme poverty and stressful circumstances" (McKenna 2005: 142), including problems with substance abuse among adults. The AAP and many physicians seem to take a "better safe than sorry" approach when formulating these recommendations, since they assume it would be more difficult to control other risk factors, including parents' alcohol, drug, or even tobacco use, but in McKenna's view, the simplistic mandate against co-sleeping could potentially increase the risk of SIDS; it can also jeopardize the nursing relationship, for which on-demand nursing and night nursing are often needed to keep up milk supplies. Tomori et al. (2016), in an ethnographic study that followed eighteen families in the United States who intended to breastfeed for two years (from the second trimester to a year post-partum), found that

> None of the families planned to regularly bedshare prior to the birth of their child, yet nearly all families did so at least periodically during the first few weeks, and nearly half of the families continued to share their beds for some part of the night throughout the year. These arrangements were driven by infants' need to breastfeed. Infants did not easily sleep on their own; they often fell asleep at the breast, only to awaken when put down in a bassinet or co-sleeper. Often, infants would only be soothed by breastfeeding, initiating another cycle of breastfeeding, falling asleep, putting the baby down, and awakening. Bringing infants into bed enabled mothers to breastfeed while also getting rest, and was particularly helpful for mothers who had a Cesarean section, which limited their mobility, and necessitated complex coordination of feedings between partners. (2016: 181)

As babies move beyond the infant stage, the risk of overlaying goes down considerably, yet the instructions to not co-sleep continue from healthcare providers. With toddlers, the risk of co-sleeping is often presented by healthcare professionals as more of a developmental one in terms of the child's emotional and psychological independence.

Co-sleeping practices become something that many EN parents practice but feel is taboo to mention to healthcare professionals. Most of my interviewees and many people online mention that they practiced co-sleeping at some point. Regarding EN in general but specifically co-sleeping, Deanna, who identified as multiracial and was forty-two at the time of our interview, nursed her son for over three years. She told me

> I started lying to them honestly or just not mentioning stuff—which is kind of terrible, but very true. Like co-sleeping. They were so worked up about co-sleeping. Bro, that's the only way we're going to rest. You know, we did it for, like, a year and a half.

Deanna's approach of "lying" to her son's pediatrician mirrored that of many EN parents who learn from not only their own experiences but often through consulting with other healthcare professionals (if they have access) or asking questions in online support groups.

Deanna also described an incident in which her son's pediatrician told her she needed to wean right away when she found out he was eighteen months old. The pediatrician said that her son no longer needed it and that *she* was the one who needed it. Deanna worked in professional contexts related to public health and felt strongly that the pediatrician's advice was problematic. She decided to seek advice from a lactation consultant and nutritionist at that point.[1] The lactation consultant was supportive of child-led weaning and gave her "talking points" for her next appointment. She told me that the lactation consultant helped with "things the doctor shoots down. But I should be able to talk to the doctor, right?" This last question speaks to the need among EN parents to be able to have an open conversation with healthcare professionals, but a fear of disclosing details about EN can hinder this type of communication. Deanna's experience was mirrored in hundreds of posts online about pediatric encounters.

Pediatric Dental Issues

The pediatric dentist's office is the space that seems to be the most frequently written about in EN support groups online (based on my observations). On-demand nursing and especially night nursing, in which the child falls asleep nursing and nurses a few or several times during the night, are the chest/breastfeeding practices that are construed by some US dentists as leading to dental caries, brittle teeth, and other serious dental health issues in young children. EN parents in online groups frequently describe interactions in which, when their pediatric dentist finds out that a parent is practicing EN and night nursing and has a dental problem, the dentist does not delve deeper into other possible etiologies (causes). In some posts and comments, dentists and hygienists would tell EN parents they needed to wean even in the absence of dental problems or before they had even looked at the child's teeth. Two of my in-depth interviewees discussed dental health but did not consider it to be a reason to wean early. Melissa, who was tandem nursing her two youngest children (age four and two) at the time of our interview, said that her older children (with whom she also practiced EN) did not have dental problems, but her youngest children did:

> I think our pediatrician said, "Well, you know, if they, if they breastfeed to sleep, then when they're done, just kinda wipe their mouth out with a cloth." Like, that's not going to wake them up.

The last sentence was sarcasm, considering how unrealistic this idea might seem to most night nursing parents. She and I discussed other factors that might be related to these problems, and she said:

> I think some of the issues that my younger children have with their teeth are genetic. The dentist said that it's something with the enamel not forming during pregnancy. Maybe. So, that obviously doesn't have to do with breastfeeding.

Deanna mentioned that her son, weaned at age three, had "one, maybe two cavities" but indicated it was nothing serious, whereas her niece, who was weaned much earlier, at eight months, "has got a face full of those silver caps." Michelle, who weaned her son around age two and a half, said that her son's pediatric dentist had mentioned EN as a "risk factor for tooth malformation" but did not say that she needed to wean early for that reason.

From my auto-ethnographic experience, my in-depth interviewees' experiences, and anecdotes recounted on parenting sites and EN groups, it was apparent that EN and night nursing do not always or necessarily translate to dental caries or dental problems. However, serious dental problems do arise among some EN children, and after reading many accounts of dentists' authoritative statements about EN and dental problems, I was interested in exploring this in more detail. A common theme in stories in online support groups about dental problems is that some pediatric dentists, rather than suggesting a solution that would allow agency of the lactating parent and child to practice child-led weaning, will suggest abrupt weaning as the only correct course of action. On these posts, people mentioned that they were made to feel ashamed when their child was found to have one or more cavities. Parents said that dentists and dental hygienists would sometimes make claims about studies showing the relationship of night nursing to dental caries, but they would also repeat popular beliefs about EN that have been discussed throughout this book, such as "it's just for comfort at this age," and "you're only doing it for yourself anyway." There were posts and comments saying that dentists told them that breast milk was no different than or that it was worse than drinks like juice and even soda for teeth and that breast milk pooling in the mouth at night has the same effect as other drinks (formula, cow's milk, or juice), which are associated with "bottle rot," or severe caries in children who fall asleep with a bottle or sippy cup in their mouths.

The following is a retelling in which I have distilled and merged information from dozens of posts and comments that typically follow these posts related to dental care and cavities in EN online support groups:

> Just returned from the children's dentist, and my three year old has several cavities. I am feeling devastated. They asked if she takes a bottle to fall asleep, and I said, no, but we are still night nursing. My daughter wakes up to nurse several times during the night. The dentist said I need to wean as soon as possible! I am SO upset as I didn't think we were close to ending our breastfeeding journey, and I know weaning won't be easy at this point. Both the dentist and the hygienist acted shocked that we were still nursing. I left in tears, feeling like the worst parent ever. When I told my partner, who already is ready for us to wean, he just said we need to follow what the dentist said.
>
> Help! Does anyone have experience with this?

Sample Comments

- That's awful that you were shamed like that. Check out [website] and share this with your dentist.
- Breast milk alone does not cause tooth decay—please get a second opinion!
- Get another dentist! Your dentist is not up to date on the latest information about this. See [website or link to article]
- I night nursed two kids for a total of seven years—not a single cavity!
- This happened to us, and I wound up weaning—it was really difficult, but I didn't know how to refute the connection to night nursing given the location of the cavities.

- My dentist said the same after a dark spot appeared on my son's tooth around two years ago. I looked up some of the information online that shows there are genetic and other factors involved. We found another dentist who was supportive and recommended [x], which worked well for us.
- Have you checked for [different physical issues, such as lip tie or tongue tie, genetic conditions involving shortened ties (or frenula) in the mouth that can result in pooling of food or drink[2]]?
- Do you wipe her teeth before bed? Also, if she drinks juice or eats other sugary foods during the day, this could be the real cause.

It is common in comments for people to post their own anecdotal experiences of their EN child or children never having cavities despite years of night nursing. These comments generally include a statement that night nursing must not be the culprit or at least not the sole culprit of tooth decay. As a participant observer, I would also sometimes comment on my own experience in a similar way. My son did not develop any cavities during the five years of night nursing; he has only had one cavity in the decade or so after that. We did not particularly excel at cleaning his teeth when he was an infant or toddler. Once we started to introduce solid foods at six months, we did try to brush his teeth after the last solid food meal of the day and before night nursing to sleep, but I never felt like we did a thorough job of brushing or that our son was also not skilled or thorough in brushing and flossing when he was little.

Some people post comparative experiences—for example, having more than one child who night nursed for several years, with one child having cavities and other dental issues and the other child with none. With these comments, the intent seems to be to show that other factors might be at play in causing cavities and that those who have these issues are not "bad parents," as they have been made to feel by dental health professionals, but instead is it "bad luck" or "bad genes." However, this can be frustrating to parents whose children do have problems and are seeking help.

As in the sample comments I include above, it is common for people to suggest possible variables that, either combined with night nursing or independent of night nursing, could cause dental caries in children's teeth. These factors include the introduction of solid foods in general, the interaction of sugary or high-carbohydrate foods or drinks with breast milk (with many mentioning the typical US diet as a culprit), dental hygiene practices, genetic factors, issues related to the microbiome (of lactating parent or child), the presence of lip or tongue ties, airway issues, medication (including antibiotics) taken by the gestating parent during pregnancy, acid reflux, pH levels in the child's saliva, and more. Some discuss protective factors (such as the presence of lactoferrin in breast milk) as the reason that it is not the "breast milk" causing cavities. Others in online support groups and other social media pages will post links and resources to information about chest/breastfeeding and dental health, which I also found useful in trying to view this topic through different lenses, including those of EN parents and of dental healthcare professionals in the United States.

Another common theme in online groups is that it does not make "evolutionary sense" for EN to cause serious dental problems, since it was practiced throughout most of human prehistory. As an anthropologist, I had also assumed that dental caries was not an issue (or at least less of an issue) prior to the origins of agriculture and the introduction of high-carbohydrate diets. That generalization seems to hold up in the paleoanthropological record, as there is much less evidence for caries in prehistoric hunter-gatherer populations than in agricultural ones (Adler et al. 2013). However, there are also dietary variations among different foraging societies in the past or present that might increase the risk of dental problems. Humphrey et al. (2014), in a study of adult teeth (dated to between 15,077 and 13,892 years ago) from hunter-gatherers inhabiting the Grotte de Pigeons site in Taforalt, Morocco, found tooth decay in 94 percent of adult teeth, which they attribute to their diet that consisted of "highly cariogenic plant foods." Among contemporary foraging societies, there is extensive variation (both across different societies and within societies) in terms of diet, contact with agricultural societies, and other external impacts on their health and environment. Among the contemporary Hadza in Tanzania, for example, dental problems among women were related to agricultural village life, while women "residing in the bush eating a diet of mostly wild foods exhibited the best oral health overall" (Crittenden et al. 2017: 12). However, men in the latter category (Hadza foragers) had higher rates of caries than those living in village settings, which the authors attribute to the fact that men and boys consume greater amounts of wild honey than girls and women.

Existing peer-reviewed studies point to a complicated relationship of human milk, chest/breastfeeding practices, and dental health. The idea that "genetics" may be responsible for why some children who nurse on demand for many years, including night nursing, has support in the scientific literature, but even given potential genetic susceptibility, environmental factors will still play a part in dental health outcomes (Vieira et al. 2014). A recent study (Shungin et al. 2019) identified correlations between self-reported dental health problems and other diseases that are believed to be heritable traits. The idea that "breast milk alone" does not cause cavities is also more complicated than it appears, as in practice "breast milk" does not exist as a lone substance, and there is no uniformity in either breast milk composition or in the circumstances associated with nursing. Hunt et al. (2011: e21313, 2) note that "the origin of bacterial communities inhabiting milk is unknown," but they suggest that the nursing relationship itself may provide some clues to how certain bacteria populate the saliva of both lactating parents and nursing children and that might also impact breast milk composition. For example, since "retrograde flow back into the mammary ducts occurs during suckling," they suggest that bacteria present in infant saliva could "provide an ideal route for the exchange of bacteria from the infant's mouth into the mammary gland" (2011: e21313, 2); in their study of human breast milk taken from sixteen samples of mothers in the Pacific Northwest of the United States, they found *Streptococcus mutans*, the bacteria that is highly associated with the development of cavities, to be present at different levels in all of the samples. Silva et al. (2019) tested colostrum (breast milk that is produced in the first days post-partum) in forty-three samples (from women in Brazil who had elective C-sections) collected before the infants had begun nursing, which decreases the chances of "external contamination" from mouth-to-skin contact; they found *S. mutans* in only 16 percent of their samples, and they found that it was more likely to be found in lactating parents who said they did not have regular dental care.

Fungi of the genus *Candida*, which can cause thrush and yeast infections, can also damage tooth enamel and contribute to tooth decay. In a study comparing breastfed and formula-fed, bottle-fed children in Brazil, Zöllner and Jorge (2003) found that the prevalence of *Candida* was twice as high in bottle-fed infants than in breastfed infants who had also never had a bottle or pacifier. The authors note that breast milk has enzymes that protect against *Candida* proliferation. However, some parents who practice EN do use pacifiers sometimes and pump milk to bottle-feed their infants, so this could be a factor in tooth decay in their children.

Trongsilsat et al. (2020) demonstrated that in a comparison between human breast milk from a small sample (n = 6) of donor mothers nursing children between the ages of five and twelve months in Thailand and samples of different types of formula, human breast milk had "low biofilm acidogenicity" and "limited biofilm formation," meaning a presence of a film of bacteria and microbes on teeth surfaces that was low enough that it did not present a risk of dental caries. These authors suggest that, "the possible reason of ECC [Early Childhood Caries] in breastfed children is possibly related to another sugar component from other source of food which accumulated in the dental plaque especially for improper cleaning children [sic]" (2020: 62). Nardi et al., in a systematic literature review of studies published between 2010 and 2020, found that several factors seem to be correlated with variations in and changes to the oral microbiome of the child. In addition to how infants were fed, these factors include how the child was delivered (vaginal vs. C-section) and other circumstances of delivery, such as "maternal exposure to disinfectants and antibiotics during delivery" (2021: 12).

The AAP includes the statement on their website: "Children who are breastfed experience improved dental health," which seems very concise and straightforward (AAP 2021) and may apply to the majority of breastfed children, who are weaned before one year, but it does not necessarily address EN and night nursing. Matee et al. (1994), in a study of 2,192 children in Tanzania who were between the ages of one and four and were nursing, found a correlation between night nursing and enamel hypoplasia, which was also correlated with higher incidences of severe dental caries. A study in Pelotas, Brazil (Peres et al. 2017) included a longitudinal study of over 1,300 children from infancy to age four and included interviews with parents and dental examinations. In this study, they attempted to control for sugar consumption in the diet. They did find an association with chest/breastfeeding beyond twenty-four months and increased risk of cavities and severe dental caries before age five. However, the recommendation of these researchers is not to discourage EN but to suggest that parents brush their children's teeth before bed with a fluoride toothpaste.

Hallonsten et al. (1996), in a study that included a detailed study of 200 at eighteen months old, found a higher percentage (constituting statistical significance) of children in the group of "prolonged" chest/breastfeeding with dental caries than those in the non-chest/breastfed group, but they also said that they found the presence *of Streptococcus mutans* and a record of a "cariogenic" diet among all the children who presented with dental caries. Weerheijm et al. (1998), in a study of ninety-six children in the Netherlands, found that among children who nursed at night, dental caries was more frequently associated with lower use of fluoride toothpaste. Patel et al. (2018) note the relationship between an infant or child's "oral physiology" (e.g., lip ties or tongue ties) can affect how a child nurses and can in turn increase the risk of dental problems.

A group of dentistry and pediatric researchers (Iida et al. 2007) examined data from 1,576 children from the (US-based) National Health and Nutrition Examination Survey (NHNES). The survey contained data from household interviews as well as health data on the children, including results of dental exams. Based on this data set, there was

> no evidence that breastfeeding or its duration are independently associated with an increased risk for ECC, S-ECC [severe early childhood caries], or a greater number of decayed or filled tooth surfaces among children ages two to five years in the US. (e950)

This study was looking at data based on dental outcomes (in two- to five-year-olds) but included children who could have weaned well before age two, and this NHNES data did not contain information about night feeding. In this study, the researchers found an association between maternal smoking and early dental caries, and families living below the poverty level were more likely to have children with ECC and S-ECC. More recently, Chiao et al. (2021) also accessed NHNES information from 3,234 children between 2011 and 2018; this was one of the few studies that specifically looked at data from children who nursed for two years or more. They also did not find a correlation between nursing duration of chest/breastfeeding and ECC or S-ECC, "even when accounting for sugar intake" from sugar-sweetened beverages (2021: 279).

If it can be accepted that multiple factors are involved in the presence of dental caries in young children, there is still a question of how this information can be used productively by dental healthcare professionals without shaming or blaming parents for things like their diet, the child's diet, the type of delivery they had, or antibiotics they were prescribed or given. Also, what steps can be taken if the parent and child want to continue with EN, including night-nursing and child-led weaning? Comments in online EN support groups indicate that there are dentists who are interested in finding solutions to serious dental concerns without forcing weaning before parents and children are ready or without drastic, invasive procedures, such as drilling or root canals that involve anesthesia, which many parents online expressed concerns about for their young children. Some mention examples of both "regular" and holistic dentists (who typically look to broader aspects of everyday living and health to understand more about dental health) offering and providing solutions that do not involve weaning or excessive and invasive procedures. The use of silver diamine fluoride, which is used to halt the development of caries, was mentioned as an effective treatment. This can cause teeth to turn black, which some parents wanted to avoid, but others felt since the baby teeth would fall out eventually, this was not permanent, or they were less worried if the black teeth or teeth with darkened spots were on back teeth that were less visible. Others mentioned things like re-mineralizing toothpaste, vitamins and supplements, changes to dietary choices, and changes to dental hygiene habits.

In reviewing online narratives in support groups, the risk of dental issues with EN or night nursing was not something that was expected or anticipated by parents. As EN and night nursing are often believed by EN parents to be the "natural" way of feeding children, it seemed counterintuitive to many EN parents that it could cause health issues. For those whose children do have severe issues, whether they are related to EN/night nursing or not, online support groups were helpful with resources, and there are examples of healthcare professionals who seek solutions that allow parents and children to maintain agency related to nursing.

Obstetrician-Gynecologists

A common recommendation that nursing parents hear from their OB-GYN if they find out they are pregnant with another child is that they need to wean because of the risks of miscarriage, early labor, or insufficient nutrition being delivered to the fetus if a gestating parent is nursing during pregnancy. OB-GYNs will cite the contractions that take place during chest/breastfeeding that can supposedly cause spontaneous miscarriage. Although nursing while pregnant can be difficult and painful for some people, some parents prefer not to wean during pregnancy and plan to tandem nurse. I will include more about the challenges involved in tandem nursing in Chapter 7, but here I wanted to focus on how the biomedical encounter can play a part in the decision to tandem nurse or not. Among my in-depth interviewees who continued to nurse one child during all or part of another pregnancy or beyond, no one mentioned being advised to wean because of pregnancy, although as noted, most were either confident about their decisions and able to inform themselves about this topic or decided on their own to wean because of the discomfort. In online support groups, in comments responding to questions about whether their OB-GYN was correct or not, participants would often post information from the LLL website that indicates that chest/breastfeeding while pregnant (in most circumstances) is safe. Sometimes people would write something to the effect that "orgasms are known to cause the same kinds of contractions, but doctors don't tell you should avoid sex or masturbation during pregnancy."

Joseph Molitoris (2019), in a study involving analysis of data from the National Survey of Family Growth, found that in over 10,000 pregnancies in the United States, that although there was an increased risk of miscarriage for those who practiced exclusive breastfeeding of an infant during pregnancy generally (when compared to formula-fed infants), there was no increased risk of miscarriage in pregnancy among parents whose infant had begun complementary foods, which are usually introduced between four and six months. This suggests that chest/breastfeeding infants who are also consuming solid foods and children beyond the infancy stage (beyond a year) does not seem to increase the risk of miscarriage. In a study in Iraq, researchers found no evidence of a higher risk of miscarriage among chest/breastfeeding women (over a range of women's ages and when compared to a control group of non-chest/breastfeeding women). In their study, which included 215 in the sample group and 280 in the control group, there was actually "a significantly lower frequency of miscarriage among those who breastfed during pregnancy compared to those who didn't," and while they found that preterm deliveries were slightly more common among the chest/breastfeeding mothers, the difference was not statistically significant (Albadran 2013: 288). In online posts and comments, some people will suggest that doctors will try to protect themselves by making a general recommendation that weaning is necessary during pregnancy, when it is only people in certain risk groups who need to do this to avoid miscarriage. If true, this reflects a common theme in biomedical encounters of healthcare professionals deciding on a blanket recommendation to wean without looking at the nuances of existing research.

Medications and Procedures

During the course of EN, which can be a few years to decades (for people who practice EN with multiple children), it is inevitable that most people will be prescribed a medication or that they or their child will need to have a medical procedure. One participant in in-depth interviews mentioned forgoing a medication that she felt might have benefited her because her physician told her it could show up in breast milk, and though she was skeptical, she chose not to take the medication rather than choosing to wean. Another (whose story with breast cancer is discussed in this chapter) weaned her son earlier than she had planned because she had to undergo chemotherapy; in this case, she and her physicians were on the same page with the decision to wean, though there are some alternatives to weaning with chemotherapy; if a lactating parent wants to resume nursing after chemotherapy treatment, they could "pump and discard" their milk to keep their supply up (Peirce 2016: Online).

In online support groups for EN, people often sought advice from others about the biomedical advice they had received about contraindications for taking certain medications while nursing. This is a distillation of many similar posts on this topic:

> I need to have surgery and am expected to receive general anesthesia and then pain medication for several days following the surgery. My child is three and still nursing through the night, with no signs of being ready to wean. My doctor said I need to stop nursing for a day (or altogether) before the surgery. Can this be right? Has anyone been through this?

Posts like this typically generate dozens of comments, which included experiences that other people in the group have had with safely continuing to nurse after surgery or while taking certain medications, and many commenters will discuss the idea that it is a "myth" that parents have to stop nursing because of certain procedures or medications or even that they need to "pump and dump" their milk before resuming chest/breastfeeding. Some comments will also include links to sites (for example, the National Institute of Health's "Drugs and Lactation Database" [NIH 2022]) that indicate what medications have been shown through peer-reviewed studies to be safe to take while chest/breastfeeding.

For children's surgeries that require fasting or clear liquids only before the procedure, there are disagreements among healthcare professionals about whether or not breast milk is considered a "clear liquid" that would not cause complications during surgery. It might seem trivial to ask that a child refrain from drinking breast milk for several hours before surgery, but when night nursing is common and a parent attempts to refuse milk, it can result in stress and tears that could also put the surgery in jeopardy. Helen Lauro, an anesthesiologist and clinical professor of anesthesiology, writing about whether recommendations about fasting before surgery should be amended to allow ingestion of breast milk or formula closer to the time of surgery, noted that breast milk "is not a complete solid," though different medical institutions classify it as clear liquid and others see it as "between a clear and formula," as a solid, or as formula:

Traditionally anesthesiologists are taught the NPO after midnight rule (Latin: Nulla per os or "nothing by mouth") from their first day of residency. Under this rule, children were lumped together with adults, and fasted for all solids including milk and clears, for eight hours prior to surgery, because of concern for aspiration. The period of time that a child can safely fast has been reconsidered in the past years. (Lauro 2003: Online)

I include her commentary here because it speaks to problems with a "one size fits all" model of biomedical recommendations as well as to how these rules that medical students learn "from their first day of residency" stick with them. As with other recommendations discussed in this chapter, there is also a lack of understanding of the lived experience of EN for parents and children, coupled with a lack of effort (in some cases) on the part of biomedical professionals to investigate alternatives to simplistic recommendations for weaning, or in this case, fasting.

Breast Cancer and Diagnostic Testing

Recent studies indicate that chest/breastfeeding confers significant protection for the lactating caregiver against breast cancer (Stordal 2023), but this does not mean that nursing prevents breast cancer in all cases. On breast cancer related posts on support groups related to this topic, members practicing EN often write that their doctor told them they can and should wait until they wean to get a mammogram. Considering that some people practicing EN are nursing beyond the recommended age to begin these screening procedures, and some may be at high risk before they turn forty because of their genetic profile or family history, a blanket statement to "wait until they're done" could put people at a higher risk of late detection. One of my physicians recommended waiting to get a mammogram until several months after my son was weaned. I was told that the results would look "weird" and could result in a false positive, and she told me that nursing provides additional protection anyway, so I waited until I was almost forty-three to have my first mammogram.

Shelby, a white woman from the Southwest, with whom I interacted through private messages after contacting her about a social media post, said that although she did get a mammogram when she was still nursing her daughter, the experience was terrible. The technician was not informed in advance that she was still nursing her child (who was three at the time), and Shelby said that the technician responded in a way that made her feel deeply embarrassed. She also had to go in for a follow-up mammogram because they had a hard time reading it, and she did. She told me in a PM:

> I was viewed as some sort of degenerate or insane mother for even going past two! But I just followed my gut and went with what I felt my child needed. And it worked. There was no trauma to the process and when we were done we were both ready. She has never sucked her thumb or had to have a comfort object because I was there for her.

When we were in touch about her post, she said her child eventually self-weaned, but because of this negative experience, she had let several years pass without going back for another mammogram. Her experience also led to further fears about disclosing to others that she was nursing. She told me, "I don't tell ANYONE this. Only her dad and I know that I didn't fully wean until her fourth birthday."

One of my interviewees (who was also someone I knew before my research began and whose pseudonym I am leaving out here for confidentiality purposes so as to not associate her with other aspects of her story) developed breast cancer while practicing EN, which prompted her to have to wean her son instead of allowing him to wean at his own pace. She had participated in different parts of my study over several years, first through messaging related to one of my posts on a social media site, private messaging, and then through a formal, in-depth interview. She told me:

> I got over three years [in, with nursing my son]. I feel like they [her breasts] did their job. Somehow, I'm ok with [the prospect of a mastectomy], because, you know, at least they had a good run, so somehow, I'm okay with it.

We talked about the fact that chest/breastfeeding is supposed to provide some protection against breast cancer, but she said she believes that she would have gotten cancer either way. After her diagnosis, she found out more about a history of breast cancer in her family, and she said that still, she believes that EN "probably staved it off for a while for a long time, honestly."

A year after my interview with her, I messaged her and learned that she had completed chemotherapy, but cancer had spread to other parts of her body. She died just a month after our last communication. Her death caused me to reflect on whether, despite the protective advantage it might provide physiologically, EN could increase the risk of late breast cancer detection for some people because of the delays that it might create for detection through mammograms—or rather, that the biomedical community's protocols surrounding chest/breastfeeding women could increase this risk. She was only forty-one when they detected breast cancer and she had to wean at that point, but perhaps a mammogram at forty could have saved her life. I am not sure if she had a genetic factor that put her at a higher risk than others for breast cancer, in which case her doctors could have recommended screening while nursing. Maybe they did, but this was not a question I asked during conversations and interviews with her, and now I cannot ask her. However, her situation, Shelby's story, and my own concerns about the recommendations given by my gynecologist to delay my first mammogram until I was done nursing made me want to look into this issue further.

Recommendations about whether or not lactating individuals should get a mammogram are not necessarily a product of popular beliefs about nursing but about incomplete information and knowledge gaps among healthcare professionals (though reactions of revulsion, as Shelby experienced, are certainly informed by these popular beliefs). The results of mammograms performed on people who are lactating might be more difficult to read, according to many recent sources, but it is possible and safe for most people who are nursing a child to get mammograms, ultrasounds, and biopsies. Citing a study by Carmichael et al. (2017), LLL recommends that women who are under thirty with the BRCA (BReast CAncer) gene, which indicates a higher risk for breast cancer, should not have screenings. The reasoning in the study is that for people with this mutation, there could be an increased risk for radiation-induced breast cancer with frequent screenings. However, these researchers note that despite the protective factor that nursing is known to provide against breast cancer and breast cancer mortality, screening is important for people in this high-risk category who are over thirty, which would include a large number of women who might be nursing children. Screening can be done through X-ray, MRI, or ultrasound. A LLL informational document includes the recommendation to ask a radiologist "who has experience reading mammograms of breastfeeding women" (2024a: Online) to read the X-ray or otherwise conduct the procedure. My impression from observations of online comments in support groups is that it is uncommon for radiologists to have this training. Pumping or nursing right before the procedure for a better read is also recommended (LLL 2024a). In an article establishing an ABM protocol for mammograms for nursing parents, Johnson et al. (2020) recommend regular screening for women if they plan to nurse for more than six months and are in a risk group or age range that would typically be expected to be screened. Shelby's experience in getting the mammogram also suggests the necessity of further training for both physicians and mammogram technicians, whose negative reaction to chest/breastfeeding parents or parents practicing EN could also provoke avoidance of future diagnostic visits.

Positive Medical Encounters

Meg, in the quotation I featured at the top of this chapter, was talking about a negative interaction with an "on call" pediatrician, but she also noted, in a PM, that she felt fortunate that her "regular pediatrician never made any sort of negative remark toward breastfeeding my son. And we stopped just past three and a half years." In this chapter, I have thus far focused on the negative incidents and iatrogenic harm, but there are positive stories of support as well.

Some of the most positive interactions that people described in online posts were from healthcare professionals who had personal experience with EN. Tami Ross (2024), in ethnographic research on caregivers for teens with POTS (Postural Orthostatic Tachycardia Syndrome), found that they had the best experiences in hospital and clinic settings when a healthcare professional was familiar with POTS, not just from a clinical perspective but from personal experience. However, personal, lived experience does not have to be/should not be the only way a healthcare professional can understand the perspectives of EN parents. Open-mindedness and a willingness to listen and learn from patients can be equally important. Several of my in-depth interviewees talked about being proactive about seeking healthcare providers who would support them in their parenting decisions. Paige mentioned that with her second pregnancy, she "wasn't vibing" with her OB/GYN, who she had heard make negative comments about the LGBTQ community, in a rural area of a Southeast US state, so she sought "the only person of color on staff . . . We both had purple hair, she came in with like purple eyeliner, and I was like, oh yeah, this is my person." Paige is white, but she took these aspects of her OB/GYN's identity and self-presentation to mean that she might be progressive and open to different perspectives. Although this physician left the practice shortly after Paige's son was born, this physician supported her nursing goals, and she (the doctor) advocated for her post-birth plan that included making sure that Paige's son did not receive bottles at the hospital. Then Paige also had a great experience with her pediatrician, who never said a negative word about EN:

She thought it was great that I was able to go as long as I did. You know, she said herself that she was not able to be that successful, and she wishes that she would have had the resources that there are now today because she feels like she could have, could have gone far. If I ever had a moment where I was struggling with something, she was just real quick to hand me some pamphlets or pull a video up online in the pediatrician's room on her computer for different holds to try to like, make him latch a little bit more comfortably . . . She was concerned he might have a lip tie, but . . . she was really advocating to not [do any invasive procedures] and try other methods and so she was really helpful, by also acknowledging that she's like, "I did not do this for very long, so we're gonna learn together."

This approach of learning from and working collaboratively with a patient contrasts with traditional biomedical interactions in which the authority typically rests with the biomedical professional.

Similarly, Caitlyn did not receive pushback from physicians, and one interaction she described with a pediatrician illustrates the fact that many healthcare professionals who are not familiar with EN are willing to learn:

I think that the pediatrician asked one time. I think she [Caitlyn's daughter] was like two-ish, and [the pediatrician] just said, you know, "Are you still breastfeeding?" And I said, yes. And she said, like, "What does that look like?" And I was like, "well, it looks like this." And she's [Caitlyn's daughter] standing up just wild, and I was "yeah, but she also is like asking for it, and I'm okay with it." And that was the last time we ever talked about it.

Caitlyn was living in a progressive city where physicians tend to be relatively open-minded, and her pediatrician's question seemed to be more about curiosity and learning with no judgment attached. At the same time, the pediatrician's lack of familiarity with what it might "look like" to nurse beyond two years indicates that EN is not generally covered in the process of pediatric specialization in the United States. It is also an indication that many pediatricians themselves grew up not seeing EN; for those who had children, often neither they nor their partners practiced EN. In these cases, for open-minded physicians, they often learn from their patients (or parents of their patients).

Nia had a positive experience in which she had a supportive healthcare professional who inspired her to become one for others in the future. She said when her son was an infant "everyone" (her family, doctors, her pediatrician) told her to "just put him on formula," when she was struggling to initiate nursing.

However, she remembered "this random lady" she had met through the WIC program[3]; she called her, and this woman did a home visit:

> She helped me and we were able to breastfeed successfully from there, only seeing her once. And then from then on, she checked up on me every few months. She helped me and then, after that, we breastfed successfully for quite a while, and she would reach out to me every couple of months to make sure I was still doing good.

Nia continued to breastfeed until her son self-weaned close to his second birthday. She talked about how this experience affected not only her relationship with her son but also her career trajectory.

> I've grown so fond of it. I loved me and my son's breastfeeding time together, and I had to reach back out to see, like, like, pick her brain a little bit, but she was [no longer working there].

Nia pursued her interest in helping others with chest/breastfeeding and after training as a doula, focused her graduate social science research on this topic, received her IBCLC, and went on to a nurse-midwifery program.

Increasing Support, Reducing Harm

> ... biomedicine makes available awesome tools and techniques for resolving certain problems of certain bodies, [but] its curative might is bounded precisely by the limits of the technical and of the particular practitioner. (Ashe 2021: 256)

This observation from Leah Ashe suggests the importance of understanding that biomedical professionals may not have all the answers and carry their own biases to their practice of medicine. EN is not an illness in need of a cure, but it is a bodily practice (affecting not just the lactating person but also the child or children who are nursing) and thus is often entangled with biomedicine. A theme that emerged regarding the experience of parents practicing EN and their encounters with healthcare professionals is that their instructions or recommendations about weaning are a combination of knowledge gaps that are often reinforced or filled in with preconceived ideas about chest/breastfeeding in general, EN, and child-led weaning. In cases where US biomedical professionals are drawing on published research or AAP recommendations, they often fail to understand the nuances of these recommendations, if they are familiar with them at all, and many people in online groups report that healthcare providers will give advice that contradicts existing biomedical data. In some cases (e.g., with dental issues and EN), a limited number of studies and sometimes conflicting data in existing publications can lead practitioners to give advice to "just wean." den Kreps and Kriner (2020) have noted that the absence of clear scientific data related to health and disease generates additional doubt and confusion and lends itself to the development of popular models. They present an example from the Covid-19 pandemic, during which information coming from government and medical authorities seemed to shift rapidly as new studies were conducted and presented to the public. I have observed the same phenomenon with Hansen's disease. There is still "scientific uncertainty" about Hansen's disease transmission and factors related to susceptibility, despite it being one of the oldest diseases known to humankind; this uncertainty also encourages people (including healthcare professionals) to fill in information with what makes sense to them, based on experience or based on the limited information they have heard. Similarly, there have been very few studies done on chest/breastfeeding beyond two years. Many studies about SIDS and about medications, alcohol, and other substances that might be passed from a lactating parent to the nursing child are focused on infants and toddlers. Children who are practicing EN but who weigh three to four times more than an infant and who get most of their calories from food will not be affected by substances that come through a lactating parent's breast milk in the same way that an infant will, and older children will be less at risk of overlaying during co-sleeping than an infant or small toddler.

I have only scratched the surface of examples from people in online groups of challenges that people practicing EN face in their interactions with biomedical practitioners, but I have tried in this chapter to focus on some of the most common perceived conflicts that arise in these settings. I am not arguing that chest/breastfeeding or EN should ever be privileged over vital or life-saving medical care or diagnostic tests for children or for lactating parents. There are certainly circumstances in which nursing cannot continue safely. However, based on the experiences of people I interviewed and whose stories I observed and collected in online spaces, there are many examples of healthcare professionals suggesting weaning without researching alternatives. As illustrated above, in some cases, weaning is suggested or mandated simply because healthcare professionals are uncomfortable with or unaccustomed to seeing or hearing about older children who have not yet weaned, whereas in other cases, healthcare professionals suggest a medical reason for weaning which indicates they may not have been exposed to updated guidelines.

There are also examples of healthcare professionals who, even if they are not familiar with the experience of EN, are willing to work with parents and learn from them or do additional research to accommodate them or help them continue with chest/breastfeeding if desired. For future research, it would be interesting to compare changes in healthcare professionals' attitudes toward EN in recent years, with the AAP updates to recommendations and as new generations of healthcare professionals themselves either practice EN or are open to learning from their patients—to revisit the quote from Paige's son's pediatrician, who was supportive in helping Paige establish and maintain her nursing relationship for as long as Paige was comfortable: "We're gonna learn this together."

6

"Cease and Desist"

Legal Issues and EN

When I began this project, I was interested in how my experience with EN was similar to or different from that of other parents in the United States; for the most part, the issues that came up in interviews and in online spaces overlapped with my own, but I had less experience with how EN can intersect with the law and the court system, other than dealing with jury duty notices, which is the first topic in this chapter. Some of the participants in my study and many people who post in online groups have dealt with more complicated legal issues that threatened not only their chest/breastfeeding journey but also their access to their children. Divorce arrangements and custody hearings bring parenting practices (EN and child-led weaning) that are mostly invisible into center stage, where they are scrutinized by legal professionals who often have little background knowledge about these practices. In this chapter, I will discuss how EN can be weaponized in divorce proceedings by the non-lactating parent and how other intersecting aspects of identity of the parents may play a part in a parent practicing EN finding themselves at risk of losing their child. The issue of chest/breastfeeding rights for both incarcerated US citizens and detained undocumented immigrants only came up occasionally in online spaces, but I discuss this briefly here as well.

Jury Duty

During the years that I was nursing my son, I received two jury duty notices; both times, although my son was no longer exclusively nursing, he was still nursing on demand every few hours and would not drink milk from a bottle. I called the courthouse to ask about accommodations for pumping or to have my husband bring our son up during breaks for me to nurse, which they said was not possible; both times, they agreed to defer my service. I understand and take seriously the responsibility of jury duty and was not trying "to get out of it," as I have seen suggested on some general parenting sites (not EN pages or groups) where people ask about jury duty and childcare. I considered being able to nurse a child on demand until they are weaned to be a human right for both him and for me and was prepared to defend this as a right, but I never faced any major challenges to my ability to do this. However, the reality in the United States is that EN and child-led weaning are generally construed in American society as privileges and not rights guaranteed by law, and in legal contexts, a parent's autonomy to make decisions about jury duty while chest/breastfeeding can quickly be overridden and seem to be up to county policies or to the whims of the individual to whom you might speak when you attempt to have jury service deferred.

Online comments on a Baltimore local Fox news video news story (Cairns 2018) about the mother of a one-year-old, who asked for and was denied breaks to pump and a fridge to store breast milk after being assigned jury duty, generally reflect societal attitudes about chest/breastfeeding. In the story, the woman (Emily Schneider) mentioned having a note from her pediatrician at Johns Hopkins saying she was still nursing, but the court did not accept it because her son was older than twelve months. In the video, Schneider says: "I just felt astonished that Baltimore City Circuit Court felt that it was their right to put a timeline on when it was appropriate for me to be able to provide breast milk to my son." Online comments on the news outlet's Facebook post (WBFF/Fox 45 2018) with this video focused on the idea that she seemed "entitled" and that she was trying to shirk a civic duty, and that the issues she faced with jury duty were the same as those that other lactating parents face in going to work. Some people commented that they were compelled to serve jury duty in a similar situation, and they pumped in advance and brought pads to manage leaky breasts. The implication from comments written by people who had also been unduly burdened by being asked to complete their jury duty service while nursing seemed to see it as fair that Schneider should also have to endure this burden. However, there were some commenters who were supportive and did feel that the expectations of the court were unreasonable.

Jury duty for nursing parents was a topic that also appeared on several US-based parenting groups I followed on Facebook during my research. There were always a mix of stories and opinions, with examples of the flexibility of some county court systems in offering a deferral and/or providing an area for the nursing parent to pump and store milk during the day. On these more general parenting groups, there would be many parents who exhibited a judgmental approach to answering the OP's question, including statements like those found on the story about Emily Schneider in the example above, in the vein of "this is an important civic duty. Why are you trying to use your child to get out of it?" This may illustrate a lack of understanding of how milk supply can be affected and the pain (and infection/mastitis) that can come with engorgement if pumping rooms are not available. Some in online groups noted that they had to get a letter from their pediatrician or another doctor or that a notarized medical affidavit was required for them to be exempt from service, which might be fairly simple for a parent nursing an infant but more complicated for someone practicing EN, depending on the beliefs of medical professionals about when weaning should occur. In some counties, juror questionnaires will ask if you are the primary caretaker for a young child, and you can check this box to be able to defer. I found it interesting that in online stories about jury duty experiences or exemptions, there was variation even when people dealt with the same county courthouse, indicating the arbitrariness of decision-making by representatives of the court, which can cause undue stress for nursing parents.

Custody and Visitation After Divorce or Separation

In my observations, the most commonly discussed legal issue related to EN in online spaces has to do with parental custody and visitation rights issues after separation or divorce. In addition to numerous posts on custody issues and divorce in EN support groups, I found support groups online that dealt specifically with court issues for nursing parents. This is an important topic; it affects so many children and families. For example, according to 2014 US Census data, over a quarter of children under twenty-one in the United States lived "in families with only one of their parents while the other parent lived elsewhere" (Grall 2016: 2). The two most common concerns that were discussed in online groups were that overnight visits with the non-lactating parents would be stressful for the child and/or put an end to the nursing relationship and that EN was being characterized by the other parent and by representatives of the court as harmful (and a potential reason for loss of custody or limited visitation rights). These are related legal issues, as the opinions of legal representatives on whether EN (and especially night nursing) are harmful or abusive practices affect how they will view custody and visitation arrangements.

In online support groups, there are stories of contentious custody and visitation disputes that involved one parent who was practicing EN or just nursing in the first two years of a child's life and one parent who was insisting on a visitation arrangement that involved sleepovers with the non-nursing parent. This can be a complicated issue. Both (or all) parents'/legal guardians' access to time to bond with their children is very important, and overnight stays can be a part of establishing that kind of bond; at the same time, separating a child from a nursing parent during a time that is already particularly stressful for both children and adults can add additional stress and trauma. In online groups, some EN parents have written about how overnights with the non-lactating parent resulted in their milk drying up, which causes distress for the EN parent and the child. Some of these posts are not asking for advice about legal issues, because shared custody arrangements had already been worked out, but about how to keep their milk supply going while separated from their child.

There are some existing legal resources online for parents with versions in English and Spanish, in a "Custody and Chest/breastfeeding Toolkit" (prepared by BreastfeedLA, ACLU SoCal, and the California Women's Law Center 2021), which includes a court letter template and contains information on arrangements for EN parents and for people practicing child-led weaning, though many of the recommendations in the toolkit are specific to California, which "has the strongest protections for chest/breastfeeding rights in the country" (2021: 5). Their court letter is adapted from a letter sample available online from the Michigan Breastfeeding Network (2018). Anthropologist Katherine Dettwyler also made a court letter available on her website, but as stated on her site, she is retired and can no longer provide signed copies (Dettwyler 2015). Reading so many stories written by participants in online groups about their custody rights being challenged in court because of EN prompted me to draft a version of a court letter that EN parents could potentially use. In the letter (see Appendix C), I provide my perspective as an anthropologist that EN and child-led weaning are safe practices and do not constitute a form of child abuse, and I make the point about the importance of divorced parents (and the court system) coming up with a plan together that is in the best interests of the child. I cite the work of Elizabeth Baldwin (2001), who has published several articles on legal challenges associated with chest/breastfeeding, including accusations of parental abuse against the parent who is practicing EN.

When I noticed that someone had posted about custody issues in EN support groups, I would post a comment that I have this general letter available to share via PM for no charge; usually, a few people would ask for a copy in the comments before the thread got buried. Over the years, I have shared this letter via PM with several dozen people. These online interactions occasionally resulted in me learning about their custody cases, and in a few instances, I also sent along consent forms to request to use examples from their experiences in publications. I have also tailored the letter to specific cases, and one EN parent requested a notarized version that could potentially be accepted as a more official document in court, though I have not heard that this letter made a major impact in anyone's case.

In writing about the experiences of people with whom I have interacted or exchanged online messages about their struggles with custody issues related to EN, I have had to think carefully about how to present the details about their cases so as not to provide too much identifying information. Fears about custody issues also make EN parents wary about posting anything on social media about chest/breastfeeding or sharing anything with family members through private messaging. This fear of not only stigmatizing attitudes but also legal action prevents parents from contributing to the normalization of EN and child-led weaning by feeling compelled to keep this information hidden. At times in a custody situation, the child also is made aware that talking openly about nursing is dangerous. They might hear from the nursing parent that they might not be able to continue having milk if they talk about it openly to other relatives, or they might be shamed by the other parent if they admit or discuss the fact that they are continuing to nurse. For most of the parents I interviewed or from whom I received consent to include some of their stories, by the time of writing and publication of this book, the children in question are now older and have since weaned. Still, I am including minimal information about their identities in these examples.

One woman with whom I have exchanged messages periodically over four years, since I first sent her a court letter, has kept me updated on the status of her case; her ex-husband and in-laws often brought up the fact that she was still nursing her child beyond the age of two in order to attempt to strip her of custody altogether. When he did have overnights with the child, he would repeatedly ask the child directly about nursing behaviors, and he brought up EN in court as something he felt was harmful to his child. The court wound up assigning a Guardian Ad Litem (GAL), a court-appointed representative who is supposed to serve as an impartial advocate for a child's well-being. The GAL first encouraged a deadline for weaning; later the GAL filed a "cease and desist" order to try to force the issue, which, she said, "was so hard for me because I really wanted [to do] child-led weaning, and with Covid and all, I wanted to extend as much as I could." As with many healthcare professionals, as discussed in the previous chapter, representatives of the legal system who have no experience with EN often suggest or try to mandate abrupt weaning as if it were a simple task: "Just stop nursing." However, once chest/breastfeeding is established, cold turkey-style weaning is not an easy task and can be traumatic for both the parent and the child. Meanwhile, with the divorce and with other changes in the child's life, it was a time when her child would more frequently ask to nurse.

> My friend told me that if my extended breastfeeding is the only fault opposing counsel and the Guardian Ad Litem could see, I must be a darn good mom.... It is only sad that the court and GAL pit this issue against mental issues and violent tendencies provided on a 911 police cam of the other party and finds extended breastfeeding more problematic.

A few months later, she was in touch and let me know that she fired her lawyer and, the proposed order with the cease and desist was not passed. But they did try, both the GAL and opposing counsel, to bring it up again with my current lawyer, who dismissed it as a non-issue. In general, her thoughts on this whole case were that "family law is failing us." Her experience highlighted the lack of familiarity with the idea of EN and child-led weaning in the family court system.

Another woman, with whom I have exchanged messages after she posted about similar legal issues, said that she also struggled with a GAL, who urged her to wean as well. This was particularly difficult for her son at the time, as he had health issues that caused frequent dehydration, and nursing provided him with not only comfort but needed electrolytes. Her own lawyer advised her to stop as well so that she would not lose custody. She mentioned that she was in a part of the United States where there was little knowledge of EN. She described a bullying style of behavior from her ex-husband, who had also moved to a location several hours away that required longer stretches of separation for overnight visits to take place.

One of my in-depth interviewees (whose pseudonym I am not including here in order to not link other aspects of her story to her) encountered a legal battle related to visitation issues with her youngest child a few years after my first interview with her. She was still nursing when she separated from the child's father because of domestic violence issues. She said that in the state where she was currently living, the court system's approach to custody was about giving "equal" custody rights to both biological parents—in other words, the gender roles that different parents might play, including the ability of one parent to nurse the child or the degree of parental involvement of different parents prior to the custody case, are not considered in custody decisions. Her perspective was that

> they don't care about any separation trauma—men's [fathers'] rights come first. My child hasn't even seen [the father] since she was eight weeks old, and they think it's in the best interest of the child for her to just be handed off to him unsupervised for three days straight.

In this case, she did not want to turn her child over to the father for several nights in a row because she was concerned not only about ending the nursing relationship but also about the abuse she had experienced.

The attitude of the court in her case reflects a fairly recent swing back to acknowledging the rights of biological fathers in the US legal system. Mary Ann Mason (1994) has detailed the complicated history of shifting court opinions related to custody in the United States since colonial days, during which children were viewed as the property of the father (or in the case of slavery, of the slave owner). During much of the nineteenth century, courts increasingly ruled more in favor of what they saw as the best interests of the child, though this was often focused on the "naturalness" of "mother love." This shift may have to do with more fathers among the "new urban middle class" spending less time in the home; Mason notes that although the majority of US households during that era were in rural areas, where fathers spent significant time at home, "even judges from rural areas shared this growing solicitude toward children and their mothers," so that "by the second half of the nineteenth century, courts from throughout the country . . . displayed concern for the welfare of the child and endorsed the nurturing nature of mothers" (1994: 52). Mason believes this also had to do with the "development of a uniform middle-class culture based on mass circulation magazines and books" (1994: 52).

In the 1970s, in part as a reaction to second wave feminism, the Men's Rights Movement emerged and is related to a shift in the United States toward a recognition of the rights of fathers. Through ethnographic interviews with men who self-identified as "fathers' rightists" in Canada, Bertoia and Drakich found that generally, in practice, the men were not lobbying for joint, equal responsibility and care of children after divorce; they want equal access to their children, to information, and to decision making. The individual, self-disclosed accounts reported here unveil a masculinist construction of equality that obfuscates the gendered differences and experiences of mothers and fathers. Fathers' rightists have coopted the language of equality but not the spirit of equality . . . The rhetoric of fathers' rights gives the illusion of equality, but in essence, the demands are to continue the practice of inequality in post divorce parenting but now with legal sanction. (1993: 612)

"Equal access" does not include an acknowledgment of the role that different parents might play in childcare. The current Father's Rights Movement website (2022) similarly advocates for "50/50 shared parenting," which sounds reasonable, but 50/50 is complicated to calculate when chest/breastfeeding, among other caregiving practices, create different roles with different time requirements. Since the 1990s when Bertoia and Drakich's research was conducted, some North American families have attempted to at least negotiate a more egalitarian relationship in terms of all aspects of childcare; in practice, however, in heteronormative relationships, more of the childcare responsibilities in the domestic sphere fall to women, including women who work full-time outside of the home (Glynn 2018), or to one parent more than the other.

Same-sex or gender fluid marriages often reproduce heteronormative arrangements. Goldberg (2013) has noted that the "homonormative" ideal is a more egalitarian division of household labor, but in practice, the division is somewhat lopsided. In Goldberg's systematic review of studies on same-sex couples and household labor division, she references Mignon Moore's book, *Invisible Families: Gay Identities, Relationships, and Motherhood among Black women* (2011), in which Moore describes how biological mothers in Black lesbian relationships are the ones who do the bulk of the childcare and domestic labor. In survey research with parents who identified as transgender or nonbinary (with partners of different gender identities), Tornello (2020) found there was also a desire for a true egalitarian division of labor, but in practice, it was usually one parent who did more of the childcare-related labor, and this was often the parents who "were in newer relationships, worked fewer hours per week in paid employment, and were the genetic parent to the focal child" (2020: 8). In an autoethnographic article, freelance author Haley Swenson (2024: Online) detailed her own same-sex relationship in relation to sharing household tasks and noted that despite planning for a more egalitarian division of labor in the home, "our queer, feminist household is looking more and more like our own parents' when it comes to dividing work and care."

Even for families who overtly espouse a more egalitarian ethos, typically it is only one parent who is doing a lot of the bodily labor associated with chest/breastfeeding. The other partner might be able to assist more with feeding tasks if the lactating parent is pumping. However, if the lactating parent is in proximity to a child who is practicing EN, there is high demand for milk and contact from that parent, both during the day and, if they are co-sleeping, during the night. Many parents in online EN support groups will ask for advice about on-demand feeding at night, which seems to escalate rather than decrease around age two, and parents note that attempts to have another parent or caregiver soothe a child back to sleep are often futile.

In terms of equally divided labor and time required for chest/breastfeeding, one contemporary arrangement that could make this possible is co-lactation, in which chest/breastfeeding is practiced by both parents. Schnell (2022) describes an example of a queer couple in which co-lactation reportedly worked well, with the non-gestational parent having successfully induced lactation; at the end of a one year observation period (one year after their child was born) for this study, the couple reported that they continued to "equally share breastfeeding" (648). Theoretically, with such an arrangement, in the circumstance of divorce or separation, it would be possible for nursing to continue indefinitely with both parents and the issue of shared custody that involved overnight visits would be less stressful for the child. Of course, this is a hypothetical situation to which most separating or divorcing parents would not be amenable.

An ideal visitation arrangement that truly represents the best interests of the child or children who are still chest/breastfeeding could involve at least temporary "inequality" in terms of time spent with the child; such an arrangement would be one in which parents acknowledge the complexities of different roles they might play in the lives of children at different stages in their lives. This could take many forms though it would be predicated on an amicable relationship between the separated parents and/or a court system that is well-informed about EN and child-led weaning. It might involve stepwise adaptation of overnight time for children at the non-lactating parents' residence; children can adapt to overnights but still might be interested in nursing when they are at the home of the lactating parent; if this is not interfering with custody arrangements or cutting into the time spent with the other parent, this should not be an issue at all for the courts.

Notably, in the examples of my interlocutors above, non-lactating ex-spouses/partners often weaponized the ideas of EN and co-sleeping, claiming abuse and child endangerment, and the court and child advocates had become the strong arm against EN. Arguably, there could be other factors involved in the families I mentioned, since I was only hearing the side of the lactating parents, and the non-nursing parent might feel that EN was also being used as a weapon for nursing parents to make excuses for limited custody.

I have seen examples of amicable arrangements in private EN support groups where parents have posted their concerns about overnight visits; in comments, parents will give examples of ways they were able to make overnight stays work and maintain the nursing relationship and their own milk supply, but generally this also required both parents' cooperation. On posts where people ask advice of other parents, a common suggestion is to make an agreement with the other parent that overnights begin with just one night per week or one night at a time, so there is some gradual adjustment and for the nursing parent to pump milk to maintain a supply when the child is not with the nursing parent. From comments in online groups, it is not uncommon for older children to pick up where they left off with chest/breastfeeding after a few nights away, but it can be difficult for the nursing parent, who might become engorged or whose milk supply gradually diminishes unless they are pumping fairly regularly. Another suggestion by members of online groups is to prepare children for the temporary separation by assuring them they can have milk when they are back with the nursing parent.

Night waking and nursing to sleep is common in infants and children once the chest/breastfeeding relationship is well-established, and this can go on for several years. Night nursing itself can be a red flag in custody hearings, as the AAP recommends separate sleeping areas for infants to promote safe sleeping; as discussed in the last chapter, co-sleeping and night nursing for older children do not present the same risks as they do for infants, but the nuances of bedsharing and co-sleeping dangers can be misunderstood by judges or GALs who know little about EN. The majority of children in the United States are weaned before age one. There is a great deal of variation by region and state in the United States as well. At one end of the spectrum, in West Virginia, only 19.2 percent of babies born in 2019 were still being chest/breastfed at twelve months, whereas a few states (Hawaii, Alaska, Vermont, and Washington) had over 50 percent of babies still receiving human milk or being breastfed at twelve months (CDC 2022). The likelihood of judges and lawyers being familiar with cases in which chest/

breastfeeding comes into discussions may be higher in states where more babies are being nursed for prolonged periods of time. The gender, race, and class background of judges and of all parties involved in a custody case can also play a part in legal outcomes.

One of my interlocutors noted that many judges practicing today are older men with very little personal experience of chest/breastfeeding in their own families. Her husband had held positions in the legal system, and he was influenced by the fact that his wife practiced EN, child-led weaning, and co-sleeping. She mentioned that once, in his investigation of a bedsharing death, she urged him to indicate in his report the difference between bedsharing and co-sleeping (which can also include just room-sharing or the use of a side-car bed) so as not to further stigmatize safe co-sleeping. As with healthcare professionals, having more judges and other legal professionals that have had positive personal experiences with chest/breastfeeding could result in decisions that demonstrate an appreciation of the complex nature of EN and child-led weaning.

Legal issues in divorce cases for queer (especially trans and nonbinary) parents who choose to nurse their children are compounded by the stigma of their gender identity, which on its own can have legal implications as well. In the Florida Circuit Court 2004 case *Kantaras v. Kantaras*, Linda Kantaras (a cisgender woman and biological parent to two children) attempted to gain full custody of her children after divorce from her husband, a trans man, arguing that their marriage was invalid in Florida as a same-sex marriage (since her ex-husband was AFAB). After an initial decision in Michael's favor, their marriage was voided by the Florida Court of Appeals; eventually, he was able to gain shared custody in an out-of-court settlement. Michael was additionally vulnerable in this case because he was not the biological parent, though he had legally adopted the older child (which also became an issue in the court case as same-sex adoption was also illegal at the time in Florida) (Lambda Legal 2025; GLADLAW 2025). Information about trans identity is more available today, and there is greater representation for the trans community, but there has also been significant reactionary legislation and heightened transphobia in the United States in recent years, particularly in the last year (2024) of my research. Judges' biases and lack of knowledge about both chest/breastfeeding and transgender issues can play a part in how other practices might come into play or are interpreted in custody decisions.

In EN support groups, trans and nonbinary members discussed experiences with nursing their children, but I did not come across posts discussing custody issues for these parents. On TikTok, which I joined in 2021, I started to follow a Black trans man and chestfeeding father, Tanius Posey, @transking30. I include his name here only because his story has been well-publicized, including in an article for the *New York Post* (Keller 2023). He documented his nursing journey with his son, which extended beyond his son's second year, as well as the birth of his second child in 2024, in daily posts and live sessions on TikTok. In the *Post* article, there is a screenshot of another user's comment, "That boy should be taken." Posey also hosted regular live sessions ("Lives") on TikTok, in which he interacted with users in real time and answered questions. During these Lives, comments stream past and users express support or disdain and ask questions. In April 2023, Posey posted a GoFundMe to raise money to relocate from Florida to the more progressive state of Washington, and he has since been able to successfully move. In his GoFundMe site, he wrote, "I just want to live without having to worry about my son being taken just for simply living and being trans" (Posey 2023). Rapid changes to the political landscape at the state and federal level may continue to affect queer parents in ways that cisgender parents do not typically have to consider.

Incarceration

An important legal issue that I did not have a chance to explore fully in this study is related to EN parents who have to serve time in jail, prison, or immigrant detention. Incarceration, either for short-term jail or long-term prison sentences, presents the risk of ending an established nursing relationship and affecting family relationships. Budd (2024: Online) noted that the "female incarcerated population stands almost seven times higher [in recent years] than in 1980," with over 180,000 women in jail and prisons in 2022; a disproportionate percentage of women are from marginalized groups. The nonprofit organization Motherhood Beyond Bars reported that "80% of women held in jails are mothers to dependent children" (2025: Online). A special 2021 issue of the journal *Breastfeeding Medicine* includes several articles that illustrate the lack of protection of the rights of nursing parents in US jails and prisons. Eidelman noted that "this reality adds to the myriad of negative health disparities" for women of color, who are incarcerated at "twice the rate of white women" (2021: 663). Nursing parents in immigrant detention and deportation proceedings in the United States often find themselves in even more precarious situations; in some facilities, young children are allowed to stay with their mothers, but the conditions are known to be substandard. Both in the several years before and during the second Trump administration, there have been numerous reports of the rights of pregnant and lactating parents in immigrant detention being ignored. In July 2021, ICE (the US Immigration and Customs Enforcement) issued a statement saying that ICE should not

> detain, arrest, or take into custody for an administrative violation of the immigration laws individuals known to be pregnant or nursing, which includes a year of postpartum in recognition of the time needed for infant development and parental bonding. (2025: Online)

However, this page, updated in June 2025 (though still available to view online), contains a note that this is now archived content: "This information is archived and not reflective of current practice" (ICE 2025).

Though none of my in-depth interviewees faced jail or prison time that they mentioned, in online support groups on different platforms, there were occasional posts related to EN and short jail sentences. It is likely that people who have to serve prison sentences or who are in immigrant detention facilities would be nervous about posting or asking questions on social media sites, or they would not have the ability to post, so the occurrence of nursing parents who face incarceration or immigrant detention is probably underrepresented in online groups. The types of questions that I did see were focused on either asking for advice about maintaining milk supply during a short jail sentence or reporting on jail conditions during an overnight or weekend experience in jail. In posts that I saw on this topic, lactating parents reported having to serve a short sentence in jail because they and their family were unable to pay fines owed for a minor, nonviolent offense. A few nights away from a nursing child might not end the nursing relationship, but the stress on both parent and child (as well as the family members who are caring for the child in the parent's absence) can be intense. It can also be physically painful to experience breast engorgement that comes from not being able to pump or express milk while in jail, of which there were also examples given by members of online support groups for EN. In examples I saw online, low-income status (or a lack of both social and economic capital), coupled with policies that criminalize nonviolent offenses, were factors that explain why some lactating parents risked jail time and temporarily lost the ability to feed their child on their own terms.

In a position paper (2023), the National Commission on Correctional Healthcare has acknowledged the importance of chest/breastfeeding and post-partum support and care for incarcerated women, and they provide recommendations for support of nursing mothers for the first two years. However, there are "only six states with state laws related to breastfeeding support for incarcerated people. Only one-third of US prisons and jails have any written policy on breastfeeding or lactation" (Center for Leadership Education in Maternal & Child Public Health, University of Minnesota–Twin Cities, School of Public Health 2023). Even for states with short-term policies and prison nurseries that facilitate the chest/breastfeeding relationship for infants and lactating parents in prison, nursing for as long as the parent and child would like to continue is challenging in the context of US incarceration for parents with long sentences. In the United States, there is one program in Washington state that was established in 1999; it allows "pregnant, minimum security inmates with sentences of less than thirty months the opportunity to keep their babies with them after giving birth" (National Institute of Corrections 2025). Corley (2018) did a feature for National Public Radio on this program, which serves not only to help parents maintain a close relationship with their babies but helps them prepare and transition for parenting after they leave the facility. The photos in the story show the small and clean apartment-like spaces that mothers share with their children and with whom they share rooms, though the women have to work in the prison during the day, which can limit opportunities to nurse on demand, while their children are cared for in a prison daycare. However, this program only accommodates twenty mother-child pairs in residence at a time.

Walker et al. (2021) did research on similar programs in Australia in which infants and young children can live with their mothers in prison settings:

> There are designated, and in some cases, purpose-built mothers and children's residential facilities at prisons in seven Australian jurisdictions. Upper age limits for children range from twelve months to five years. However, we found that children above three years of age are rarely accommodated. Accommodation is modelled around domestic life, with pregnant sentenced prisoners and those with children typically living in free-standing units with capacity for ten to fifteen mother–child pairs. (2021: 24)

For this program as well, there are limitations on eligibility, and the authors note that Aboriginal women they interviewed, though underrepresented in their sample, were at a higher risk of losing their children than others, often because of the multiple forms of disadvantage they faced. Walker et al. also discussed the problems with residential programs, both in terms of the experiences and rights of children in adult prison settings and the expectations for mothers, who have limited autonomy within the context of incarceration.

Spain has similar "Mother Units," where incarcerated women can stay with their children. Jubany-Roig and Massó Guijarro (2024) did ethnographic interviews focused on chest/breastfeeding experiences in these contexts. Some of the women they interviewed described challenges to establishing and maintaining chest/breastfeeding for reasons that are not unlike those of women in non-carceral settings, although several described forms of "obstetric violence," daily policing, and lack of support for lactation difficulties. In their sample, there was one woman who nursed her child for more than two years, though most of the women (of those who had weaned) nursed for less than six months.

I would argue that even the most progressive model for allowing parents to stay with their children is still problematic if it is carried out in the context of incarceration, where both parents and their children are institutionalized and have limited freedom. Reforming certain aspects of the prison system in the United States, in which many people serve time in jail pre-trial because they cannot afford bail or are imprisoned for misdemeanor offenses, is a partial solution (Sawyer and Wagner 2024). Diversion programs for people with misdemeanor and/or nonviolent offenses are one such approach; in diversion programs, people are able to continue their lives out of jail or prison pre-trial if they participate in counseling, addiction treatment, and sometimes community service activities which, if they are eventually convicted, could also reduce or complete their sentence before the conviction. Diversion programs can also include parenting and lactation courses for pregnant people or parents of small children. One such program tested by Motherhood Beyond Bars was successful in the Fulton County Jail in Atlanta, Georgia in 2024:

> In February [2024], MBB began its first diversion program in Fulton County, which is close to where the organization is based. They offer reproductive health education to pregnant individuals in Fulton County Jail while also pinpointing potential diversion candidates . . . In the first six cases where they were able to talk to the women who've been arrested, work with their public defender or attorneys, find a placement for them, and present this option to a judge and the prosecutors, [Executive Director of Motherhood Beyond Bars, Amy] Ard says MBB has had a 100 percent success rate in getting women diverted from the prison system. (Dakshit 2024: Online)

It could be argued that these kinds of programs also save taxpayers money long-term and have the potential to improve health outcomes for families and children. However, societal and political support for diversion programs or other restorative or rehabilitative programs for those accused or convicted of crimes can depend on the political climate, and as long as prisons and jails are part of a for-profit industry, there will be less support among those in power to make or fund major reforms to the system.

Takeaways for the Legal System in the United States

At present in the US legal system, there seems to be inconsistent acknowledgment, particularly in carceral settings, of AAP or WHO basic recommendations related to exclusive nursing for the first six months and for two years and beyond, "as mutually desired by mother and child" (Meek et al. 2022) or to the ABM's assertion of chest/breastfeeding as a human right (Feldman-Winter et al. 2022), with even less consideration given for the choices of parents or children to practice EN or child-led weaning. Parents who had intended to continue nursing for as long as their child wanted to or even just for the first few weeks or months of their children's lives may find themselves stripped of the agency to participate, with their children, in these decisions about feeding. Alternatives to incarceration, like diversion programs or home detention, could allow chest/breastfeeding to be established and continue. In immigrant detention centers, which are often out of the public eye in remote locations and where even the most basic human rights protocols are not being followed, the rights of chest/breastfeeding people need to be highlighted more in the media for change to take place.

The most-discussed legal issue on EN support groups that I observed over the past decade was related to visitation and custody arrangements after separation or divorce. It was clear from posts and comments that these accommodations were most likely to be satisfactory to all parties only when the relationship between the lactating parent and the parent was amicable, so that they were able to work together on an arrangement that benefited the child and all parties. When this relationship was contentious, participants in my study and others who posted in online support groups reported that judges, GALS, attorneys, and other legal authorities knew little to nothing about chest/breastfeeding and less about EN or child-led weaning, and sometimes these legal authorities tried to mandate abrupt weaning. The experiences of my interlocutors indicate a need for greater training and education among representatives of the legal system on EN. At the least, if I were to suggest a policy recommendation, EN should never automatically be assumed to constitute child abuse or child endangerment, and judges and child advocates should be wary of claims by the non-lactating parent and their attorneys that nursing parents are practicing EN for their own benefit. I believe that there is room for improving accommodations for chest/breastfeeding or EN parents and their children without infringing on other parents' rights to access to and bonding time with their children.

7

Lived Experiences of EN

I think after all these kids, I really didn't expect it to be so much a part of my life as it has been, but I don't think I would do it any other way.
—Melissa, practiced EN with four children, including tandem nursing two of them

"Lived experience" refers to the personal experience of daily life from the perspective of the person who "lives" it. For parents who practice EN, chest/breastfeeding plays a significant role in their daily lives for many months, years, and even decades (for those who practice EN with more than one child). In previous chapters, I have focused on how the experiences of parents/caregivers practicing EN have been shaped by their interactions with others in both negative and positive ways. All of these interactions are also part of the lived experience (or lived experiences) of people who practice EN, but in this chapter, I focus more on the EN experience beyond the comments and preconceived ideas that others espouse, which include many aspects of the daily realities associated with nursing a child beyond infancy and into early childhood that are not expected or included in what most people learn growing up in the United States. These realities often result in first-time EN parents changing their own preconceived ideas about chest/breastfeeding, sleep, and parenting in general.

For people who have access to social media support groups or other virtual groups in the contemporary context, these unexpected experiences are shared and validated in support groups online. For many people practicing EN, no other spaces exist to tell stories about EN that would seem strange, unbelievable, and certainly "out of place" to outsiders. Although there are in-person breastfeeding support groups like LLL, as nursing children reach a certain age, it becomes less common to find peers in one's social circles who are open about nursing children beyond age two or three. Online groups in particular serve to normalize and validate aspects of EN, at least among people who practice this who might otherwise have thought they were alone in their experiences. I found that in-depth interviews and additional interactions (via PM) or Facebook comments were also validating for me and helped me understand, from both personal and academic perspectives, more about EN beyond my own experiences and beyond the published literature on the topic. I also tried, through my interviews and in participant observation in online spaces, to share my perspectives and stories with others. In this chapter, I focus on some of the challenges as well as some of the humorous and interesting aspects of people's daily lives while practicing EN.

I begin with a discussion about how many EN parents do not necessarily plan to practice EN, but once chest/breastfeeding is established, weaning becomes more complicated. This is followed by sections on other aspects of EN that many parents did not anticipate, including nursing while pregnant and tandem nursing, on some unexpected physical aspects (which could be perceived as challenges or just interesting realities) of EN, and on navigating how older children verbalize or otherwise communicate their need to nurse as they get older. I include a discussion of the logistical and practical aspects of chest/breastfeeding and EN while making a living. There is a section about how lactating parents perceive health benefits of EN for themselves and their children and how the Covid-19 pandemic affected parents' thoughts and practices related to weaning. I conclude with a discussion of how EN parents represent their lived experience in online spaces through humor, memes, art, and milestone badges, as well as how they choose to commemorate the years they spent engaged in chest/breastfeeding.

The Unexpected Duration of EN/Child-Led Weaning

In Charlotte Faircloth's (2013) ethnography about intensive parenting in the United Kingdom and France, *Militant Lactivism*, many of the women she interviewed in her ethnography were intentional about "intensive mothering" (a term first coined/described by Sharon Hays [1996]), based on an attachment model of parenting that also constructs this as the most natural way to raise children. EN is intensive because of the time and physical/emotional commitment that it entails, though I would argue most forms of active parenting are "intensive" in different ways. Although many of my in-depth interviewees did plan to nurse their children for a specified time (usually one year or two years) they had learned was "optimal" from public or global health organizations or research, and some followed an attachment parenting style, most expected that self-weaning would take place earlier or would be easier to do.

Tomori et al. (2016) had similar findings in an ethnographic study with low-income women in the United Kingdom who nursed their children for different lengths of time; they also found that most participants who nursed "long-term" also did not plan to nurse for as long as they did. One of her interviewees said that it was "just a gradual thing that happen[ed] . . ." and "I never could have imagined breastfeeding a four-year-old child," comments which "demonstrate that they had not envisioned themselves continuing long-term" (182). Andrews (2022), in research on chest/breastfeeding mothers in Norway, also mentioned that a mom who practiced EN for three years had "unconsciously drifted into the practice" (63). Dowling and Pontin (2017) also found that in research with EN parents in the United Kingdom, most did not plan to nurse for as long as they did.

As children get older and continue to show no signs of self-weaning, many parents felt like they were entering unknown territory. They often did not expect, for example, that a three-year-old might still be waking to nurse in the night every few hours or that their seven-year-old might continue to ask for milk here and there and show no interest in giving it up altogether. Many also did not expect that they themselves would, despite these challenges, want to continue nursing a child for as long as they did, because of the observed and perceived benefits or because they felt active weaning would be more stressful for them and their children than continuing.

Deanna had initially expected to nurse her son for about a year but continued for several years. Deanna's mom nursed her, so she said there was not really a question about nursing her son and was fortunate to not have a difficult time getting it started. She thought of nursing as:

> the thing to do, like, if my body is going to make it, I wouldn't seek it out elsewhere. I don't know, it just seemed like there was never a question. Even when I was a baby, you know, a little kid thinking about having kids, I always [figured I would breastfeed].

After a year, she realized it would not necessarily be easy to wean. She said, "he didn't like bottles and even if you put breast milk in bottles, he would just wait for me to get off work, and he would just hold out all day, you know?" I knew from experience, as this happened with my son. In the first few weeks of his life I was pumping milk and giving my son a bottle, but after he (and I) got the hang of nursing, we stopped using bottles, and I returned my breast pump. When I had to go to work, he refused bottles, so my husband started to bring him to my campus office so I could nurse between my classes. This "bottle refusal" is not uncommon in breastfed babies and presents challenges for those who work full-time and do not have as much flexibility at work. Maxwell et al. (2023), in an article with the excellent title, "Why Have a Bottle when you can have Draught?" noted that although bottle refusal

> has received surprisingly little attention in the literature . . . [h]undreds of thousands of references are made to it in global breastfeeding groups, parenting forums and on social media with an emphasis on the negative impact of bottle refusal and, in turn, requests for advice on how to "solve it." (2023: 2)

Once children are beyond infancy, they are supplementing with solid foods, but there is still a need for them to drink milk (or formula) several times a day, and if they cannot/will not drink from a bottle, it becomes complicated for nursing parents to be away from their children for any length of time until their child can drink from a cup.

One of the most difficult parts of EN for me, particularly as my son got older, was that he relied on my milk to fall asleep. In over five years, we only spent a few nights apart. Despite a strong feeling (shaped by my background in anthropology) that EN was not harmful, as my child got older, I wondered if self-weaning would ever take place. A friend to whom I mentioned night nursing challenges said once, "it sounds like the 'breastaurant' is open 24/7," which felt very true. In the last year or so of nursing, it was rare for my son to ask to nurse during the day, but he still nursed frequently at night.

For me and for many of the people I interviewed or observed online, weaning was mostly "gentle," a gradual process of negotiation between the nursing parent and the child. There were some who decided or were compelled to take a more active role in weaning their children—sometimes because of divorce or custody issues or medical reasons, as discussed in previous chapters; challenges related to work; a need to travel independently; and/or discomfort, which took many forms—for example, physical discomfort or more psychological discomfort which could be exacerbated by pressure from others to wean. For those who did not face these issues and wanted their child to truly lead the way, weaning sometimes took place well beyond the age they had expected it to happen. Among in-depth interviews, four and a half was the longest nursing duration at the time of interview, but in online support groups, I saw numerous posts about nursing children who were older, up to nine years old. Posts about children self-weaning between the ages of five and eight were fairly common. At this age, people often note that nursing is very infrequent—often just once or twice a day or a little bit at night to fall asleep. I have seen several posts over the years about EN and children who are neurodivergent or autistic. Many parents write about EN as helping greatly with children's emotional regulation as children get older. There are also posts and comments about self-weaning taking longer with special needs children primarily because their children relied heavily on nursing to feel soothed; for the most part, this was discussed in a positive way, with parents commenting on how nursing helped their neurodivergent or special needs children find calm in difficult situations.

"Child-led weaning" suggests the agency of the child, but there is also quite a bit of agency in the decision of the lactating individual in how and when to let a child/children nurse from their breasts. Even when a parent has made a conscious decision to practice child-led weaning, there are many unconscious actions that the lactating parent takes to discourage on-demand nursing or to increase the amount of time between feedings. As children get older, the lactating parent and the child might spend more time apart, and in some cases, this also leads to gradual weaning. I gave my son a lot of agency in access to nursing, but I also did small things that led to him weaning earlier (maybe) than he would have if given full agency. When he was three, we got him his own bed (in his own room); after that, I would still nurse him to sleep in his room and then leave after he fell asleep. Sometimes we would stay up late reading, or I would say he could have milk after I sang a long song (like "100 Bottles of Beer on the Wall"), and (sometimes) he would fall asleep before I got to the end. I took advantage of the fact that I was leading a study abroad program in Brazil in the summer after he turned five. We would often go out with my students at night and stay up very late, so that when he did nurse, he would fall asleep within a few minutes.

The number of times in a day (and during the night) that children beyond infancy want to nurse was also unexpected for many who practice EN. Since most EN parents also practiced "on demand" nursing when their children were infants, they were familiar with the fact that babies nurse often and on their own schedules, unless a strict schedule is imposed on them. Many parents thought that nursing would become far less frequent once solid foods were introduced and once children no longer relied solely on breast milk for nutrition. However, it is not uncommon for children who are two or three years old to ask to nurse multiple times throughout the day—sometimes it might be just for a few seconds before they are distracted by something else, or it could be multiple, longer nursing sessions each time they wake up in the night.

Some of my interlocutors also took subtle steps toward weaning when they started to sense their own discomfort, though kids were not always on board. Kim said when she was ready to gently wean one of her kids, she would tell her daughter, "okay, but just for a minute, or just for ten counts," but "she will put her hand over my mouth. She'll be, like, 'don't count, mommy!'" Melissa's youngest daughter was two years and four months old when I interviewed her. She said she had started

> doing little things to maybe get her less dependent on it. So, like, we'll sit in [chairs next to each other] where I'm on the computer, and she'll be watching a YouTube video . . . [she'll nurse while] watching her video, and I'll kind of start to turn the chair and so that she's trying to, like, stay attached. And then she gets, she's just "whatever, it's too much trouble." And so she pops off and that's about the extent of [that nursing session].

Melissa's story mirrors that of other stories I saw on EN and gentle weaning support groups online, in terms of using distractions to gently discourage uninterrupted attachment to the breast, which, over time, can lead to weaning more rapidly than unlimited access.

Others might take more active steps, like going away for the weekend and leaving the child with the non-lactating parent or other caregiver or throwing a "weaning party," with much discussion leading up to it, to celebrate the "last day of nursing." There are also many children's books written to help children conceptualize an end to the nursing relationship, though many of the extant books (e.g., Reid and Zepeda [2021] and Guy [2022]) are geared more toward toddlers rather than to the experience of older children (over four) who are nursing and whose parents might want to take steps to wean.

Birthdays are often milestones that parents talk about with children as the "coming of age" point when nursing will or might end, as these are generally recognizable as rites of passage for children as they get older. During our interview, Sam said that she was no longer producing much milk, so it had been mostly "dry nursing" for a while:

> She still asks to nurse, and we still give it a go and every now and then she gets a little teaspoon of milk. [Her daughter will ask:] "Will it work tomorrow?" I had this conversation this morning. Yeah, actually she said, "well, when my birthday comes, I won't nurse anymore." And I said, "and then my milk will go away," and

she said, "oh, how does it go away? How do you explain that to a three year old in the morning?"

For Nia, changes to habits during the day and transitioning her son from co-sleeping to sleeping in his own bed helped with gentle weaning:

> I think it started during the day. Throughout the day, if we were busy, I just would tell him "later," and so eventually we dropped down to only during . . . at night or for nap. I really wanted him to be out of my bed, and I felt kinda intuitively that I was a distraction in the bed . . . I wanted to really transition him to get [to the point where] I could put him in his own bed, because I felt like he would sleep better and he did, or we transitioned. So I kind of got him really excited about being in his own bed, and breastfeeding just kind of went away. No fuss really over it. It was super gentle. It probably could've continued if I wanted to.

She also mentioned that in co-sleeping, when he would fall asleep, he would grind his teeth, which sometimes resulted in him biting her accidentally and also contributed to her feeling like she was ready to wean.

In interviews and in comments and posts I saw in online spaces, it was clear that even for parents who chose child-led weaning, they had underestimated the extent of what "extended" would mean in terms of time and emotional labor. Still, they perceived there to be more positives than negatives, and when parents had practiced EN with one child, they often planned to practice it with another child. Among my interviewees, the only regrets expressed were among those parents who said that they did not or were not able to allow their child more agency in weaning because of external factors, including pregnancy, as I discuss in the next section.

Nursing While Pregnant and Tandem Nursing Challenges

Some participants in interviews and many in online support groups wrote about how nursing more than one child at once was not planned. Often, people expected that the older child would "naturally" stop nursing if their nursing parent was pregnant. Pregnancy frequently makes nursing more painful or uncomfortable, which often leads to more intentional weaning on the parent's part, and the taste of breast milk can also change, so some children wean themselves at this time. Sugarman and Kendall-Tackett (1995) in survey research with 179 women who practiced EN, also found that pregnancy was one of the reasons weaning was not fully child-led among their sample.

Ashley said that she weaned her oldest child at age two and a half, "because I was pregnant, and it started getting uncomfortable." Richa said that she also wound up taking more active steps to wean her first child when she was pregnant.

> I was still nursing her through the night, and it was exhausting . . . we did the Pantley [Elizabeth Pantley method], whatever, no-cry sleep solution where you pat her back to get her back to sleep. And it took a couple of months, but that sort of led to daytime weaning . . . so she didn't ask for it as much during the day. I had a little bit of guilt that because I was pregnant with him, I had to make her stop, and maybe she wasn't really ready to, but in the long run, she's fine. I met my goal of two years. I didn't feel like I had the strength to tandem—I didn't think I had it in me, so that's what put the fear in me to try to stop.

Her son (and last child) nursed for almost four years though. For many, the last/youngest child was the one more likely to nurse for the longest time since there was not another pregnancy involved that could complicate chest/breastfeeding.

Some nursing relationships persist throughout the lactating parent's pregnancy; other children might be temporarily weaned during the pregnancy, either because the child stops liking the taste and self-weans or because the parent is uncomfortable nursing while pregnant, but when milk comes in after childbirth, the older child might ask for it again. Anne had this experience with her older daughter, who was four when Anne's son was born:

> I think I had this idea in my mind that I would wean her when I was pregnant, and I did have my supply drop. I think more towards the beginning and then it was also [really painful] so I did struggle a little bit, but she was so adamant about wanting to continue. At that time, she was sleeping in her own bed but I would nurse her down and just kind of lay with her while she fell asleep. So we went through that process where she would sleep on her own, and then when the baby [their second child] was born, she wanted to nurse full time again. So anyway, all that to say, it sort of just ebbed and flowed with what worked.

Melissa practiced EN with four children but struggled with nursing through pregnancy and with tandem nursing, though she practiced the latter with her youngest two children after more actively weaning her oldest child during her second pregnancy. She recalled:

> I thought I probably did not want to tandem nurse. [My daughter] was almost three when [my son] was born and so. And I think I did, I must have. I nursed a little bit during pregnancy. Let's see . . . I think at that point, I was kind of ready

to sort of encourage her to wean. Like, I wasn't going to just cut her off, but I did try to like, say, "Okay, we're not going to do it out in public. Okay now we're only going to do it, whatever. I don't remember exactly how I did it, but I really wanted her to be done before he was born . . . And I remember it being kind of difficult and lonely because, you know, she had been sort of co-sleeping a lot. It's hard to remember that far, but she did, she did eventually quit before he was born.

However, with her two youngest children, she said:

They're closer in age. My son had just turned two when [my youngest] was born. And I thought maybe he would stop, because I really felt like I had dried up during my pregnancy, but he, he was all in. [This was during] the pandemic; she was born in [the fall] of 2020. And I remember it being really painful and uncomfortable during my pregnancy and I really hoped that he would quit but there just wasn't a way to wean him, you know, and I didn't want to before he was two. Then once she was born, oh, he was all into it again. Because you get all that newborn milk, and he wanted to be on me all the time. When she was nursing, he wanted to be there. I would have to kind of like discourage him a little bit, because it seemed like he was getting all the milk before the baby could, but, you know, he got to be very vocal, and it was, he loves it so much and it "tastes like strawberries." I don't know why he would say that but [laughs].

Ultimately, she also "cut him off" when he was three years and eight months old, though he still was not a "willing" participant in weaning at that time. She said it just got to be too much to handle, especially in terms of sleep, and as happens with many nursing parents, as will be discussed further below, she said:

Generally, when they become toddlers, I sort of to begin to develop a little bit of an aversion because the way a toddler nurses feels different, and, like, the way their teeth are on your nipple is different . . . so it was really affecting my mental health.

Melissa nursed children for the longest total time (about eleven years altogether) of any of my interviewees, but she also took active steps to wean when it became uncomfortable and untenable. Her quotation that opens this chapter indicates that the major role of chest/breastfeeding in her life was unexpected, but she also talked about being able to "learn over time, like, you know, with different kids, to have so much knowledge." This speaks to the point that this generation of parents who are practicing EN are, for the most part, gaining knowledge from their own experience or through online sources, rather than being able to draw on generations of practices they learned or were exposed to as they were growing up.

"Gymnurstics," "Twiddling," and Other Quirks of EN and Sources of Nursing Aversion

Sarit Guy, who nursed five children and practiced EN, wrote and illustrated three children's books about breastfeeding that show the nursing relationship and can be used with young children to both celebrate chest/breastfeeding and facilitate gentle weaning. In one book (*Mommy's Hug—Weaning from Breastfeeding Together*, 2022), there is an illustration of a child with one leg sticking out to the side with the other leg between the mom's legs, in sort of an acrobatic type of pose. The text on this page has the child saying:

> From time to time, I still nurse, and do a little trick. I nurse and stand on one leg. Look, mommy, quick! Sometimes, I tickle my mommy, or tease, or move from one side to the other with ease.

In online support groups, there are numerous posts about children's nursing positions, and some people will post photos of their children nursing in a number of different positions—for example, upside down and standing over the nursing parent or standing next to the parent and nursing while the parent is on the computer. Much of the discussion in private groups of these positions serves to provide commiseration among parents who sometimes tire of, but are also amused by, nursing children's antics and acrobatics, and in Facebook private groups especially, people will mention that they would "never post" about this on their personal pages. These "gymnurstics," as they are often called, and nursing while standing up or while being engaged in other activities, reflect how comfortable children are in the nursing relationship, but they can be seen as "out of place" in the wider society. A *Time* magazine cover from 2012, along with the accompanying, polarizing story ("Are You Mom Enough?") (Pickert 2012), that generated much controversy when it first came out, featured a standing woman nursing her three-year-old son while he is standing up (on a stool). Although the *Time* photographer posed the mother and son in this way to be provocative, knowing that some would see the position as odd or obscene, this position is very typical of the experience of nursing an older child but is also something with which many Americans are still uncomfortable.

In contrast to the privacy that some seek in private support groups online, on public Instagram, YouTube, and TikTok accounts, some users/creators will share photos and videos/reels of their children nursing in positions that contrast with the stereotypical image of chest/breastfeeding, one of an infant or small child at rest in a nursing mother's arms. There are accounts that feature photos and videos, for example, of a parent doing yoga positions while a toddler is standing up or sitting down and drinking milk from one of their breasts. POV (Point of View) videos of EN, of which it is possible to find hundreds using hashtags or search terms like "extended breastfeeding," "tandem nursing," "extended chestfeeding," "breastfeeding a toddler," and more, give viewers an idea of what it looks like to nurse a squirmy toddler or to nurse a larger child or to tandem nurse children of different sizes/ages. There will usually be a series of negative comments on most of these videos. Most of the videos on TikTok, notably, are of people filming in their home or another private space; of course, the internet is a very public stage, but comments received in online settings may feel safer than comments or actions that EN parents are concerned others might make/take in the "real world," as Claytor (2021) pointed out in a thesis about people who come out on TikTok while remaining closeted to their families. The stated goal of creators is often to "normalize" EN, while comments suggest they are only doing it "for attention" or "clout" (likes, subscribers, etc.) and that they are harming their children.

My interlocutors were supportive in theory of normalizing public nursing, and some said they did not care what others thought about it. Others were more cautious, especially as their children got older, and wanted to protect themselves and their children from stigma. In addition to using "code words" related to asking for milk, as discussed in the next section, many people found ways to be discreet about nursing children who can run/walk/stand in public. I tried to avoid nursing in public, mostly because of anticipated stigma about EN. I remember being increasingly hesitant to share this information that I was breastfeeding as my son got older. However, there were some circumstances where I also needed to nurse in public settings. On overnight flights when my son was three, four, and five, he mainly nursed at night but was still dependent on nursing to fall asleep. I would attempt to cover us both up with a blanket or wrap, but I felt very self-conscious.

Kim also talked about the difficulties of covering up during an airplane flight with her three-year-old:

> I feel awkward myself, like, if we're on a plane and she's nursing, right? . . . and she's raising my whole shirt if she's nursing and one side of her head kind of blocks what's being [exposed] . . . She's tiny. That's good. She's only 30 pounds. But even still like, she's still three feet tall, you know, so on the plane, I'm like trying to angle her feet in and, you know, things like that. Because when she's on your lap, like, her head is here, her legs are out here. She doesn't just fit in this frame anymore.

She talked about how her daughter seemed relentless about access to her breasts sometimes:

> There'll be like, oh, great advice, like, "wear a sports bra," [but] unless I straight up strapped them down with the bandage, there is nothing that child couldn't get into. I don't care—turtlenecks? Yeah, she'll put her head down a V neck with no trouble.

Although awkward nursing positions and pulling on clothing can be irritating for nursing parents in private contexts/at home, they are made doubly uncomfortable by the perceived need to "cover up" so that others cannot see a child nursing and to conceal related behaviors in public settings. Deanna talked about how her child's size, even when he was a toddler, played a part in her not wanting to nurse in public:

> He's a head taller than everyone in his class because his dad is. So, I think they would be like, you see his long legs and people are like, "That big ol' boy, you need to put him down, blah, blah, blah."

In *Breastfeeding Older Children*, Sinnott (2010) also noted that she and many people who responded to a questionnaire about EN said that they did not practice public nursing as their child grew and also did not disclose it to people generally. Dowling and Pontin have suggested that this lack of disclosure of EN as children get older could contribute to the "invisibility of long-term breastfeeding" (2017: 69). However, as my interviewee Ashley stated, even if you are an active supporter of parents' rights to publicly nurse your children, "You just don't want their looks. . . . [you don't want] that battle every day."

Other physical aspects of nursing an older child can lead to nursing aversion for EN parents involving inadvertent sensations for the nursing parents. Sociologist Pam Carter reviewed some of the literature on breastfeeding and sexuality in her 1995 book, *Breasts and Breast-feeding*; she noted then that the global health literature from the late twentieth century often ignored sexuality altogether in publications on chest/breastfeeding; some scholars tried to point out that there was no connection between breasts and sexuality, while other scholars asserted that breastfeeding was part of a "unique female sexuality" (Carter 1995: 135–40). More recent, and less gender essentialist, interpretations point to both biological and cultural origins of an association of nipples with pleasurable sensations. Using "fMRI" (functional magnetic resonance imaging) of the brain, Komisaruk et al. demonstrated that nipple stimulation (in their study, self-stimulation) can "activate the genital sensory cortex" (2011: 2828). During milk production and nursing, the hormones prolactin and oxytocin are released as well, which can cause uterine contractions and a feeling of well-being as well as involuntary orgasm in some cases. This is a topic that is complicated to bring up, mainly because there is the danger of augmenting the stigma associated with EN or with chest/breastfeeding in general. Polomeno (1999) suggests these positive sensations generated during chest/breastfeeding are something that could be explained, from an evolutionary perspective, as contributing to a longer term nursing relationship. These phenomena, coupled with the societal emphasis on the sexualization of women's breasts in the West, as discussed in Chapter 2, can make EN more complicated for parents.

In private EN groups online, the topic of arousal associated with nursing is brought up in a post occasionally; comments are invariably very supportive and generally along the lines of this being a physiological response related to oxytocin release or other hormones that are released during milk letdown. Many often mentioned feeling "icky" about it but also emphasized that it is not a reason to feel shame. On social media, I have also seen posts and comments suggesting that the aversion that sometimes comes about with EN may have to do with embodied guilt about arousal. Sinnott (2010) included a section in her book on participants who wrote about arousal during chest/breastfeeding in response to a questionnaire about EN. She said that "were at pains to stress that any arousal experienced was not directed toward the child in any way" (2010: 160). She noted that some categorized these feelings as "sensual" rather than sexual; this distinction is a way for parents to distance themselves from possible stigma that could arise in discussing these sensations.

Another phenomenon that some people in online support groups have commented on is what seems to be arousal among children, particularly erections among infants and toddlers during nursing. This can make parents question whether there is something wrong or whether they are doing the wrong thing by continuing with nursing, and it can contribute to nursing aversion as well. Posts about this topic are generally followed by a number of responses reassuring that it is normal for an infant or toddler with a penis to have an erection, and that it is not really a sexual response. Commenters point out that erections among boys can happen easily, including in simple activities like a diaper change, but this can become more of an issue for lactating parents as their children get older and can contribute to aversion, which is in part triggered by sociocultural views about body parts, gender identity, the limits of childhood, and concepts of sexuality.

It is also common for children, as soon as they begin to develop fine motor skills, to "twiddle" (usually gentle pulling, pinching, and twisting) the nursing parent's other nipple while they are drinking milk from one breast. Twiddling is a subject of almost daily posts on EN support groups because for most people it is both physically irritating and a source of emotional/psychological discomfort, in part because of the associations of nipple stimulation with sexual stimulation. The constant touching and pulling of this sensitive part of the body can become overwhelming and can for some be a reason to start the weaning process earlier than intended. The degree to which parents on EN support groups and in interviews for this research discuss twiddling in a negative way counters the popular perception that child-led weaning is a selfish practice that is about the lactating parent's needs. Instead, most parents who practice EN push through discomfort or try to find solutions to twiddling and other uncomfortable forms of touch, which can include repetitive motions, like rubbing the nursing parents' arm over and over or pulling on hair.

Stephanie talked about how twiddling and other things her son was doing while nursing were difficult for her:

> At the very beginning of twiddling, I had to shut that down, because I can't even—it makes my whole body [shudder]. We had a brief period of time—and I had to shut it down each time—but he does do a lot of like caressing, of the face. There are definitely times where I have to say, "Ok, one more minute." And the timer would go off. But fortunately, now [her son was two at the time of our interview], he doesn't nurse that long; it usually takes a couple of minutes. It's not like those [sessions] that go on and on. Cause there will sometimes be, mornings especially, where I'll bring him in bed, and he'll lay in bed to nurse like, 20 minutes, maybe longer.

Kim was gently trying to wean her three-and-a-half-year-old when I interviewed her, and she talked a lot about how twiddling was one of the bigger challenges associated with EN. Many of my interlocutors emphasized that they were looking forward to having their bodies "back" to themselves, and while many also talked about enjoying the closeness with their child, they often felt "touched out." As Kim said, "Sometimes I sit down on the couch, and I'd like to just sit there [quietly/by myself] for a few minutes without [being touched]—you know?"

On one public Facebook page ("The Leaky Boob") US-based writer and site creator Jessica Martin-Weber frequently posts questions to her followers about general issues associated with chest/breastfeeding. In one post, she included an image of a late eighteenth century Japanese woodcut by Kitagawa Utamaro that depicts a woman nursing a toddler while attempting to fix her hair. Her child is on her lap and twiddling her right breast with their left hand while reaching out for a toy that another woman standing behind the nursing woman is holding out. Martin-Weber captioned the photo, "Babies have been twiddling the other side since . . . forever!," followed by information about the art piece and about twiddling behaviors and information about gentle weaning materials she offers, while also stating, "PS: You don't have to wean to stop behaviors that annoy you, you can keep going" (Martin-Weber 2023: Online). The hundreds of comments on the post are a great illustration of twiddling as a behavior that generates discomfort or aversion in many. Several people used the phrase that twiddling "makes their skin crawl" to describe how this feels. On EN support groups, many people write that this kind of touching is particularly difficult because they were victims of nonconsensual touching or sexual abuse at some point.

Participants on social media sites I followed did not see twiddling as something that people should endure for the sake of the child. In these comments and in Facebook private groups, people regularly shared their advice for getting this behavior to stop. The most common suggestion for dealing with twiddling and other forms of uncomfortable touching is to "set boundaries," particularly when a child is old enough to understand, though if this aversion is too overwhelming, gentle weaning was often encouraged by other commenters. In comments, people suggested solutions to stop twiddling, such as holding the child's other hand, giving the child something to hold in their other hand, like a stuffed animal or a fidget spinner, or, for older children, giving them rules about touching and sometimes taking a pause from nursing to discourage twiddling. Covering up the other breast to limit access is another strategy. Interestingly, some parents wrote online about twiddling continuing after weaning has taken place, particularly in co-sleeping situations.

Nursing aversion as children get older might be compounded by gender dysphoria for people who have undergone or are in the process of undergoing gender identity transition. Creator Tanius Posey (@transking30), mentioned in the last chapter as someone who is very public about his journey and who has been featured by different news outlets in the United States, wound up nursing his first child to age two. In a TikTok video in response to someone else's question about dysphoria, in particular mentioning that it was particularly difficult when getting dressed because none of his shirts fit (because of changes in breast size related to nursing) but:

> it doesn't last with me all day long . . . because I have to feed him, and I have them for a reason and [I can] feed my child so I can't really be mad at it, but it is pretty, pretty dysphoric to me . . . but feeding and just looking at him on a day-to-day basis kind of makes it easier to get through. (Posey 2022: TikTok video)

He also mentioned how "going out" is the main issue with gender dysphoria. In this TikTok, he said that some days he chose not to leave the house at all—as a trans man with facial hair but also with larger breasts that are producing milk, he has talked about how others perceive him. For him, the dysphoria related to prolonged chestfeeding has more to do with others' reactions or anticipation of how others will respond rather than with his personal sense of identity or the nursing relationship with his children.

"When They Can Ask for It"

As discussed in Chapter 3, a common popular belief related to weaning that fits into cultural imaginaries of children's maturation and independence is that if a child can verbally ask for breast milk, they are too old to be nursing and it is time to wean. This is an interesting belief that does not take into consideration the broad range of ages in which children begin to speak. The implication in comments about "asking for it" is a verbal expression, one that can be heard by others and presumably makes others uncomfortable. Of course, "asking" for something can also be communicated in different ways. As some have pointed out in online spaces, an infant's cries or a toddler's gestures can be forms of asking for milk. However, verbal communication is often perceived (in the wider society) as a sign of maturation, which is in turn associated with the need to wean and be independent from the nursing parent in other ways.

My interviewees and people in online spaces found that when their child started to ask for milk verbally, parents both anticipated stigma and/or experienced stigma through negative comments from others, especially if children used a term or phrase that is recognized by others (e.g., "mommy milk" or "booby milk"). While some parents are unbothered by the negative attention these phrases attracted, often as children get older and are still nursing, many parents introduce a code word or gesture so that they can ask for milk without others knowing. I learned and then taught my infant son some American Sign Language signs, having read that children can learn signs before they can typically speak; my son could do the sign for milk, which is squeezing a hand like you are milking a cow, when he was about nine months old. After he knew the word for "milk," signing was a way that he could "ask for it," without most people knowing that he was asking. My son started using the word "napnos" when he became more verbal. I think it was a variation of "nipple," even though that was not a word I used often around him (at least that I can recall). "Napno," though, was a word that no one else but my husband recognized. He also sometimes just asked for "milk." On a few occasions at other people's homes, when he would ask for milk, an adult would offer to get some (cow's) milk from a cup, and I would have to explain that he did not mean that kind of milk.

One of my interviewees, Ashley, said that one of her sons used the term

> "nursie," like: "uh oh, there's a boo boo on your nursie" . . . [but] I taught the kids the word "breast" because it's anatomically correct, and I hate half of the slang terms people use [such as "tits" and "boobs"].

Kim, who was working on gently weaning her three-year-old daughter when I interviewed her in 2023, said that they use the term "nanas." Her daughter used this term "because what that's what I called it to her before she could talk, because that's what I called it with my mom, which is funny." She said that her and her two siblings "each had a different name for it, but that was mine," and she mentioned that "it can be useful" to have a term that others might not recognize as a way of asking for breast milk.

In an Appendix to her book, *To Three and Beyond*, which is a collection of narratives by women from several countries who practiced EN with their children, Janell Robisch (2014: 255–7) included a section on "Milky Names," a list of eighty-nine names that children used to talk about breasts as well as words/phrases they would use to ask for breast milk. Most are English or variations of English words with some German, Italian, and Spanish derivatives. Over the years, I also recorded terms that people in EN support groups and other nursing-related pages online mentioned that their children use to ask to nurse. Occasionally other parents on these sites would create a post with a direct question about what other children/parents use to refer to nursing—some posted this question out of curiosity/fun and others said it was because they were looking for advice, out of concern that their child was using terms that could (or had) attracted negative attention in public or at a family gathering. In these threads, many people had stories about their child or another nursing child shouting out something like, "I want boobies!" in public. I collected 174 different terms and/or phrases that children ask for breast milk as people reported online or in interviews, but there are literally infinite possibilities because of the ways children combine and create sounds and phrases. I do not include the full list here because some of the terms are so unique that they would make it possible to link the terms or phrases to individuals through an internet search. However, there were some very commonly mentioned terms, like "milkies," "milk," "nursies," "boobies," and "nanas"; most of the other terms were children's variations or alternate pronunciations of words associated with breasts and milk in English. Some people also mentioned that they introduced a term for milk or nursing in other languages, often a language that is spoken by someone in the family but that was not recognizable to most people in the United States. Like Ashley, some people online talked about trying to use "anatomically correct" words like "breast" or "nipple," but sometimes the words they tried to introduce to their children got distorted and then their children continued to say it, though it sounded like a "nonsense" word. Over the years of observing in online groups, I also saw some mentions of children who would use a click-like sound or other paralinguistic features to summon their nursing parent or to indicate that they want to nurse. Terms, signs, etc. might change as the nursing relationship evolves and a child matures, and communicating the desire to nurse could look very different for a two-year-old compared with a seven-year-old. There can be a much more secret language of asking that develops over time, but the "secrecy" reflects the wider societal stigma and also arguably contributes to EN remaining less normalized.

Practical Concerns of Making a Living/Childcare

Among my fourteen in-depth interviewees, everyone had worked full or part-time outside the home or attended a graduate level academic program full time and had to spend some time away from their children while chest/breastfeeding. They managed this in different ways, which in some cases meant switching to a different line of work that was more conducive to EN and childcare in general.

Only one interviewee, an engineer, said she resigned (at least for the time being) to be a stay-at-home mom, but this was only after her only child was already over two years old. Even for parents with a flexible schedule, like my own, negotiating chest/breastfeeding and EN while working was challenging.

For those who needed to rely on others to take care of their children, finding the right daycare was important. In a qualitative study by Schafer et al. (2021) of childcare providers in Florida, the researchers found the vast majority of providers were uncomfortable with storing or having contact with breast milk at all, expressing concerns that as a bodily fluid it could be dangerous to handle, and many daycare centers discouraged nursing on site (e.g., at pickup or dropoff). Many daycares in the United States have a policy against storing breast milk for children who are over one year (Shepard 2024), which makes it less likely that nursing can continue past this age for children who attend these daycares. Sam related a story about her experience with one Montessori school:

> We did have an interesting intersection where our breastfeeding choices in our Montessori education decision came to a head and we ended up pulling our daughter out of school. I never heard my husband raise his voice before this happened. But the school recommended that we wean our daughter at 18–19 months. What really was going on was that the teacher had had a pre-term infant and breastfeeding was very challenging for her. My daughter was very verbal, and whenever I would be at her school, if anything negative happened, she would cry, right? Because that's what toddlers do, and then she'd say, "No, I want milk." And it upset the teacher tremendously. And they said that I needed to wean or our daughter would be effectively suspended.

They left the school and, after a legal challenge, avoided the expensive cancellation fee. Sam and I talked about whether she thought this was a result of the teacher's own personal issues or part of the Montessori philosophy (which encourages children to gain independence through life skills at an early age), and how both factors may have come into play. She said the experience led her to do some research on the educator, Maria Montessori, and her philosophy of childrearing:

> [I thought], "Maybe I misunderstand Montessori. Maybe Montessori is for bottle-fed children who were off the bottle early." So I started [looking into it], and she [Maria Montessori] did have this early on "off-the-bottle" [philosophy, related] to a plan for independence but when she did studies in India, she saw that it was biologically [normal]. In Italy, she was working with orphan populations post-war.

Sam and her husband found another daycare (with a different child care philosophy) and noted the contrast:

> It was so interesting when we went on the tour. So [my daughter] was here with me, and she put her hand in my shirt, and the school director said, "She's still nursing?" and I said, "yeah," and she goes, "that's so beautiful."

Social class can play a role in whether parents have the time and income to find a daycare that will support their nursing and weaning practices.

Gabby said she took the maximum maternity leave that she could, but that was just twelve weeks. She was working as a medical assistant living in a Midwestern state. One thing that helped with continuing to nurse, she said, was that in this state, employers were mandated to give two breaks for pumping every day, and the employer "is in charge of finding a replacement [in the workplace] for when we need to pump." Also, her husband stayed home for the first almost two years:

> So nice. That was great. But, yeah, when he got a job, we had to start putting her in daycare because, you know, the hours. So he works thirds [third shifts/night shifts] and I worked ten plus hours a day. So she's in daycare now. So, she has a lot of kid interaction, which is what we wanted for her, because I don't plan on having another one for a little while.

I asked if they said anything in the daycare setting about EN, and she said that she did not run into any issues. Because her daughter was two, the daycare could give them her pumped breast milk or soy milk ("since she's allergic to dairy"), but Gabby said her daughter mostly would have breast milk once when she was at home.

Paige discussed the importance of nursing as a way to spend some quiet time with her son at the end of the workday. She was working in a demanding position for a state-level department of conservation and often had to be gone all day. She said (of nursing):

> It's really nice too cause it requires you to kind of like just sit and—kind of if you're overwhelmed, like you know you need to sit and focus on this one thing and, you know, your heartbeat I think lowers a little bit, like it puts you in this kind of like a relaxed state, like you're not thinking about multiple things at once, like your body's working right now and it was just some quiet time sometimes and also time just for me and [my son] to connect after a day, so it wasn't that he was hungry, he just like, missed me. I'm like, I missed you too—so like a way to reconnect.

Stephanie also mentioned the importance of "reconnecting" through nursing, especially at the end of the day, but she had the opportunity to see her child in breaks throughout her workday. She worked in a university administrative role and also returned to work twelve weeks after her child was born. She talked about how difficult this was, but because the campus had a daycare, she was able to go there and nurse, "sometimes once, sometimes multiple times a day. . . . That first week, I somehow forgot parts of the pump multiple times, so I'd be going over there three times a day." She mentioned that nursing from the body, as opposed to pumping, was also better for keeping up her milk supply.

Caitlyn had a graduate degree in education and was teaching middle school when she had her first child; she had fourteen weeks of leave; when she went back to work, her husband was working from home, but she said:

> I was gone all day. And we had a wonderful nanny who was coming in and helping us out and she sent me pictures around my pumping times [which can help stimulate milk production]. I had come up with a schedule—it was really tricky. My principal at the time was a man, and I went into it, like, really hard-headed. Like, "I will be pumping at ten o'clock. [Another teacher] is coming to my trailer to relieve me." I ended up having to pump in the copy room because [the trailer where she was supposed to nurse] was outside, but to walk all the way to the building, and all the way back would have added like, an additional five minutes on each side. And I was like, I'm not doing that to myself, but I really—I was really like, I'm going to make this work. I had a refrigerator in my trailer. So, I didn't have to worry about that, and I would go in the copy room and lock the door and hope nobody came in with their key to get their copies. And I would pump. And I was like, standing by the door ready to go, waiting, and if somebody was even like two or three minutes late to come relieve me, like, I was texting the principal." So I was like, "We are doing this, we will make it work," and it was hard because I missed class time, and I felt like I was doing a disservice to my students because I wasn't with them the whole time and it was hard having to have somebody come down [to sub for her] every day.

In the copy room where she had to pump, she said that "teachers would give their kids their keys and say, "go get these copies." And people would walk in. And I'd just be over in the corner with my pump." Gabriela Alvarado, a maternal health researcher with a background in family medicine and training as an anthropologist, has noted the importance of an adequate lactation room for parents who are going back to work. Alvarado's son, like my own and Deanna's (mentioned earlier in this chapter), refused to take a bottle when she had to resume work, which was fine when she was working at home, but when Alvarado traveled (with her son) to conferences, she encountered substandard lactation spaces. Her negative experience prompted her to illustrate an ideal space where lactating parents can either nurse their children or pump their milk; she included this illustration and discussion in a recent article in *Breastfeeding Medicine* (Alvarado 2025), including a locking door and spaces to clean and store bottles. Caitlyn's experience of struggle to pump in the less-than-private copy room of a middle school is one that is similar to what many nursing parents face and is a reason that many do not continue to nurse beyond a few months.

Caitlyn also talked about how she attempted to be open with her students. She had to store her milk in the refrigerator in her classroom and tell them, "this is breast milk for my baby," but she saw this as a learning opportunity for students, as she wanted them to see this as something normal:

> I would let them [her students] put, like, their Gatorade or whatever, in the refrigerator. I didn't care. Yes. And I was, like, "just don't move it," and they were like, "right, we won't touch it." And I was like, "that's great." And it was. I found the kids were much more open, much more amenable to the fact that our schedule is a little bit different sometimes because that's what was going on or that I wasn't walking them to lunch because I was going to pump in that time.

Though Caitlyn did not continue to teach after this first year of her child's life, middle school children's exposure to the idea of pumping and storing milk so that she could keep her supply up and minimize her own engorgement at work allows a younger generation to see aspects of chest/breastfeeding that are often hidden from the wider society. Caitlyn finished out the semester of middle school teaching, trained to be an IBCLC (International Board Certified Lactation Consultant), and was practicing through a private chest/breastfeeding service center when I interviewed her.

Michelle was a full-time physician/teaching faculty member, and her son was in daycare from a young age. She pumped consistently and gave bottles early on, so the transition was not as difficult for her son. She said she thought he might have preferred bottles because he could get more milk that way:

> He went back and forth just fine, and then when we, like when he went to daycare when he was three months old like, to the day, and was all bottle during the day and like, that he just—I think he just wanted it however he could get it . . . and then he would nurse [at home] in the morning and at night.

She also noted that one thing that perhaps made it possible to nurse for as long as she did was the Covid-19 pandemic, during which she wound up spending more time at home. Prior to having her child (and before the pandemic), she was traveling often to conferences and doing international research.

Work outside of the home does not necessarily preclude EN and child-led weaning, but the circumstances of that work can facilitate or complicate maintenance of the nursing relationship in many ways. Maternity leave, spaces to nurse or to pump, employer support, and access to childcare that supports EN are all things that allowed people among my interview sample to continue to nurse, often for longer than they had even anticipated, though sometimes my interlocutors had to go out of their way to demand accommodations to which they were entitled. In both online groups and in interviews, it seemed that once nursing was established, it could continue as long as the lactating parent was able to maintain a milk supply and chest/breastfeed at night or in the morning.

Perceived Health Benefits and Pandemic Protection

Studies about the short and long-term benefits of chest/breastfeeding for children are often posted and discussed in EN support groups, and these were part of the motivation to "make it" to at least two years for some of my interviewees and for many people online. However, beyond these perceived benefits about which they had read or learned, parents have their own observations of ways that EN made their and their children's lives easier. In many situations related to parenting, nursing provides a quick fix for strong feelings or minor injuries. Deanna perceived nursing and breast milk to be so helpful that she was in no rush to wean her son, despite pressure from all of her family: "It was a cure all [if] he was sad or hungry or sleepy, or you got hurt like, literally anything." She mentioned that when her son was an infant, he had a severe, extremely painful injury, and nursing helped them to get through it.

In my own experience, I felt like the ability to nurse "saved the day" for me on many occasions. As challenging and uncomfortable as nursing a child on a plane can be, for example, it was a great way to make sure my son did not experience the ear pain on takeoff and landing that is a common reason for babies and toddlers to cry on planes. On one of the study abroad programs I directed in Brazil when my son was three, my son and I both got serious food poisoning; we were alone in an apartment in Rio de Janeiro for a few days while my husband accompanied students on an excursion, and I believed nursing helped my son recover and avoid dehydration.

Having a supply of breast milk available as a home remedy for treatment of several minor ailments for which it is perceived to be effective was also something my interlocutors saw as a perk of EN. Breast milk is sometimes used as a home remedy not only for the nursing parent and the child but also for other family members and even pets. Paige mentioned saving and freezing breast milk to use for many purposes:

> It would, like, immediately clear [things] up and we still use it for [clogged] tear ducts. We used it for, like a warm bath, breast milk bath when they have really bad eczema outbreaks, it helps tremendously. . . . Ear ointment, we put some in [her older daughter's] ear when she had a bad ear infection and it helped.

Caitlyn said she used it for cradle cap (a kind of dermatitis that some infants have), and a coworker of hers mentioned using it for sunburn. I used it on my own minor eye infections frequently and found it to be quick and effective. In online spaces, sometimes parents talked about giving breast milk in a cup to older children who were sick but who were already weaned. Some of the ailments that people in EN support groups have mentioned using breast milk for include: eye infections (pink eye, styes, conjunctivitis), cuts, skin infections and injuries, diaper rash, cradle cap, acne, bug bites, sunburns, ear infections, eczema, and as a nasal rinse.

These are all examples of perceptions of breast milk's efficacy, based in part on experience, but it should be noted that there is mixed scientific evidence for breast milk's use as a home remedy. Ukponmwan et al. (2009) noted that breast milk application has been associated with serious complications or vision loss in some cases of bacterial conjunctivitis in a study in Benin; the authors dismissed the efficacy of breast milk for the more common viral form of conjunctivitis, saying that the "self-limiting nature of the infection convinces mothers that the conjunctivitis resolved as a result of the breast milk application" (2009: 32). However, other studies demonstrate that breast milk has some efficacy for eye infection (Pimple et al. 2024; Sugimura et al. 2021), and it is a common remedy cross-culturally and in different historical contexts (Baynham et al. 2013).

One of my in-depth interviewees, Sam, who was a certified lactation consultant and pediatric health coach, mentioned that her own health and her understanding of the potential benefits to health for gestating and lactating parents were some of the reasons she wanted to have children and chose to practice EN:

I think maybe it's almost selfish, but . . . I have a history of polycystic, ovarian syndrome and I know that breastfeeding helps reduce that estrogen load on the body. Full term nursing, you know, beyond the second year was going to be important for me hormonally to kind of get that under control. My grandmother also died from breast cancer . . . I haven't had the genetic testing . . . but there's a concern of what's going to happen with my reproductive organs if I don't use them in a biologically normal way. You know, are my uterus and ovaries going to continue to rebel against me? Not that I had a child as a medicine for myself [but] knowing that we wanted to have children and then finding a way to make that parenthood decision is biologically helpful for me. So that I can last to become a grandparent.

Her perspective of at least partly utilitarian way of thinking about pregnancy and breastfeeding, seeing them as contributing to her own long-term health and disease prevention, both draws on the idea of the "naturalness" of these practices and demonstrates how an awareness of the academic literature on these connections played a part in her decision-making about EN.

The perceived health benefits of nursing during the pandemic were also often discussed by EN parents. I did nine of the in-depth interviews for this project toward the end of or after the Covid-19 pandemic. I also spent a significant number of hours online during the pandemic and in the years since the vaccine has been available. At the height of the pandemic (2020–2), on social media sites, there were frequent questions posed related to Covid-19, chest/breastfeeding, and EN—to the point where on one support group, the site administrators would make announcements to encourage people to search to see if a question they were going to post had already been posted by someone else. Because of the relative lack of biomedical information about Covid-19 in general, especially in the very early days of the pandemic, many parents on the site relied on previous findings they had seen (and would share online) about how antibodies are passed to children through breast milk for other diseases. A common question was whether chest/breastfeeding should continue if the lactating parent tested positive for Covid and the child had not. For the most part, advice on the site was to continue nursing—the rationale was that since exposure had probably already taken place, isolating at that point was not going to protect the child, and antibodies were being made in the parent's milk that could be passed on and become a source of protection.

Once vaccines started to be made available to the public in the United States in 2021, there were many questions posed on social media. There can be overlap in parents who are vaccine hesitant or practice vaccine refusal and those who practice EN (Reich 2020), but I did not notice anti-vaccine rhetoric in private online groups, which may be a testament to the administrators of the groups where I spent the most time observing. Instead, people shared not only their perceptions of the protective value of breast milk but also links to the most recent peer-reviewed studies about how antibodies from the vaccine could be transmitted in human milk. On social media sites, many people who were actively practicing EN expressed feelings of gratitude that they were able to pass on additional protections to their children when there was an extensive delay between the time when adults were first eligible for vaccines in the United States (spring of 2021) versus children age five to eleven (November 2021) and under five (June 2022) (CDC 2024), though again, these feelings were something that they could not often express outside of private groups.

Caitlyn talked about being frustrated that her daughter self-weaned before she could get vaccinated:

> It took so long for the vaccines to come out and then for me to be, like, an eligible person to get the vaccine. Yeah, I was like, please do not [self] wean, please, please, please, until I know that I can get the shot, and it was just by like, a month or two, she just kind of tapered off and we were right there at that bed time and it was just, "This is not going to happen, is it?" And then then we were done, and I still hadn't gotten my shot and I was like, "dang it." Yeah, 'cause I was like, "this could have been so great." And then I've had a booster during this [current] pregnancy. So I'm like, well, this baby is like, super protected. Right? That's a good thing for this.

Melissa was tandem nursing an infant and a toddler in the year the vaccines came out, but was concerned about "losing" antibodies through nursing, an idea that I also saw voiced in some Reddit threads:

> That was one of the things I was asking about when they came out with the vaccine—can I have it when I'm breastfeeding? . . . Will it change my immunity if the antibodies are leaving my body because of breastfeeding?

By 2021, there were studies being published that demonstrated that antibodies generated by the vaccine could be passed to children through breast milk in vaccinated parents (e.g., Gray et al. 2021) though this does not result in lactating parents "losing" immunity. Discussions and links to different studies were frequently shared in online support groups for EN. During the pandemic, major news outlets—for example, *The Washington Post* (Pretzel 2022) and *The Los*

Angeles Times (Evans 2021) wrote stories about parents who were choosing to delay weaning to continue to provide immunity to their children. Both articles began with an acknowledgment of EN stigma. For example, the *Los Angeles Times* piece opened with the story of Mireya Tecpaxohitl Gonzalez, who was already "used to stares at the grocery store when she breastfeeds her three-year-old son"; this is followed by a statement of the common popular beliefs about EN: "And before you judge her: She's not doing it for attention and her kids are not spoiled because she continues breastfeeding them" (Evans 2021: Online). While it was clear that Gonzalez was already comfortable with EN and child-led weaning, she continued to encourage her older child (age seven) to continue for the perceived antibodies she could receive:

> Gonzalez was already planning to continue breastfeeding her son and 7-year-old daughter. Now, she is urging mothers to be vaccinated and continue providing breast milk to protect their kids. "We can actually talk about weaning and she's old enough to know what antibodies are," Gonzalez said. "We call them little warriors in the milk and she's willingly drinking it; she knows about the pandemic." (Evans 2021: Online)

Pre-pandemic, I also found posts online about parents waiting to wean until flu season was over. Even though children were at lower risk for severe complications with Covid than with the flu, the global panic associated with the pandemic may have made more people consider prolonging nursing.

In 2022, a major formula shortage in the United States was discussed on EN sites and on parenting pages and groups. In EN groups, many people posted about feeling relieved that they did not have to rely on formula; this shortage further validated EN for some. The tone was not gloating, but sometimes people would comment that they were glad they resisted all the pressures they had received to wean. On general parenting sites and general chest/breastfeeding pages, lactating parents who were producing an excess of milk were offering to share.

Another outcome of the pandemic was that those who were practicing chest/breastfeeding and EN had some relief from the gaze of the outside world (including extended family). Amy, whose mother-in-law challenges were detailed in Chapter 4, told me how much easier nursing was with her second child, who was born during a bad RSV (Respiratory Syncytial Virus) season (fall 2019) in which visitors were not allowed at the hospital. This was followed by the Covid pandemic, but she said nursing during this time was a positive experience because there was "no interference." The day after her maternity leave ended, Covid shut everything down. It was challenging to work from home, supervising virtual learning for her older child and nursing her younger child, but she said that the nursing part was "great" because it was done in near isolation, with no one to judge or comment and "no big family gatherings" to attend until 2022. Michelle, who had her child in 2021, also talked about how she experienced little to no stigma associated with nursing her son as he got older because she was working from home most of the time:

> You know, I think that having had a baby during Covid, we were a little bit sheltered from everything because people didn't see, you know, and it's not necessarily something they would ask about.

Although working from home was not an option for millions of parents who were classified as "essential workers" during the pandemic, many people in the United States still socialized less and visited extended family less often, which may have facilitated EN to some extent and protected people from the judgmental eyes and comments of others.

Memes and Milestones

Among those who practice EN, humor and creative artistic expression related to EN are used in daily life and in online spaces for many purposes, including to mock some of the stigmatizing attitudes they encounter from others, to represent the unexpected aspects of EN, to illustrate their own experiences with EN, and to build solidarity and a feeling of "normalcy" for others who practice EN. On social media, these forms of expression include memes, videos, anecdotes, photographs, videos, and comics.

One genre of visual representation that I noticed frequently in private support groups and parenting groups on social media is of mammals nursing offspring that are larger than most people in the United States are perhaps used to seeing. Just as in all social media spaces, cats are a popular subject. Members of private groups frequently post cat pictures as an illustration of the fact that if kittens are not removed at an early age from their mothers, they will nurse for much longer than people expect (which typically means that they appear to be adults in size, though they may be just a few months old). One post mentioned a cat that nursed for two years, and many people in comments speculate on how this might represent what offspring-led weaning would look like if humans did not interfere. I noticed a post that was made in different support groups with a photo of full-size cats/kittens that were nursing, and I followed the link back to a public page that was animal-focused and read through some of the comments there. Although there were some comments about the cats being too old to nurse, reflecting that even for nonhuman mammals, nursing babies that "appear" to have moved past the infant stage are seen as out of place or weird by many, there were also a number of comments that were a satirical play on the typical things that people who practice EN hear as reasons they should wean. For example, "those cats can already meow" (i.e., kids who can talk should be weaned), "she just wants attention," "she should cover up or other kittens will see," "get them some real milk already," "they should be drinking out of a cup by now."[1] These and similar comments (probably made by chest/breastfeeding parents) also challenge the cognitive dissonance that EN parents perceive others to have in their insistence that they wean their children before they are ready.

Posts with art from different eras that illustrate EN are also common on parenting and chest/breastfeeding social media posts and in comments. EN and tandem nursing were frequent subjects of European Renaissance and Medieval paintings, and some paintings (particularly of the Madonna and baby Jesus) illustrate behaviors like twiddling or standing while nursing. Photos of statues of nursing children from around the world are posted occasionally also. I saw photos in several groups and pages on social media of a statue in South Korea of a naked woman with two children (both toddlers or young children, standing on their own). One child is standing in front of her, ready to drink from one breast, and the other child is standing behind her (and balanced with his feet on her buttocks) and is drinking from her other breast, which is slung over her shoulder. The nursing woman has her mouth open with laughter. This statue is by Chinese clay sculptor Yu Qingcheng and is in a sculpture garden on Nami Island in South Korea (Naminara Republic 2025). LLL USA posted a photo of this statue on their Facebook page with the caption, "Is this a toddler's dream or your nightmare?" (LLL USA 2021) reflecting an acknowledgment that tandem nursing toddlers can be physically challenging, even as the mother in the statue appears to be laughing. While some commented on how wonderful this representation was, some suggested that it was asking too much of nursing parents. There is also text across the photo that says, "Breastfeeding is timeless," and it is one of several photos with this text in a series that includes paintings and photographs of nursing children in different eras, suggesting that nursing, EN, and tandem nursing were the norm across time and cross-culturally. When the same photo was shared in EN support groups online, people who comment tended to find the photo extremely relatable—funny but not extraordinary or exaggerated.

In private EN groups, participants also post photos of themselves and their children in odd positions or places, often while the nursing parent (and often the child) is multitasking. The "gymnurstics" referenced above is a common theme for these posts. There are also many posts of children wearing costumes (for Halloween or just for fun) that are funnier because the children are nursing—for example, shark or dinosaur costumes—or a mom in a cow costume.

Some of the art on private EN groups is of art or photos of art that celebrates the nursing journey. A common trend of which I have seen many examples is a "tree of life," breastfeeding image in which a photo of a child nursing is filtered or stylized so that tree roots appear to emerge from the nursing breast and a tree is growing inside the child. These are popular across nursing sites, though, and are not exclusive to EN groups. Some parents will post professional photoshoots of their child or children nursing, which can also serve as a way to commemorate the nursing journey, as I discuss more in the last section of this chapter.

Another common theme of posts in online EN support groups is related to seeking validation for and celebrating milestones associated with nursing duration. This is most notable in the posting of "badges," sometimes accompanied by stories or, mostly images of a badge and text, like "I breastfed my baby for x number of months or years." I have seen several threads in which someone will post how many days they have been breastfeeding and asked others to comment their numbers. Answers will include exact numbers, since these are fairly easy to calculate if nursing was initiated around a child's birthday; several noted that the number of days included multiple children (e.g., 3,575 days, 3 children), but it indicates the desire to further share a marker of accomplishment measured in time, much as a runner might document miles covered. The 13.1 or 26.2 (for half-marathon) on bumper stickers or car magnets are markers of pride that few would be afraid to display, but there are no comparable bumper sticker marking years or decades of chest/breastfeeding. One person commented on TikTok that she had been nursing children for her entire adult life. The need for validation and other forms of acknowledgment of these milestones is related to the fact that many parents who practiced EN do not feel like they have friends and family who would think of these milestones in a positive light, so they only post these milestones in private groups. These are paraphrasing from hundreds of similar comments or posts in private Facebook groups:

No one in my family or friend group gets it, so I wanted to celebrate this here, where I know people do understand. I'm really proud of how far we've come. I can't share this on my personal page, so I'm sharing here. We reached X years. We went through a lot to get here [examples: colic, lip tie, mastitis, other child or parent illnesses, disparaging comments from others]. Can anyone share a badge that I can repost?

LLL USA's Facebook page has a set of these badges for each month of breastfeeding through thirty-five months and then badges for three, four, five, and six plus years and "until my child outgrew the need." They also have over 300 badges, which also include references to nursing through challenges, like, "I breastfed my baby . . . through postpartum depression!" and "I breastfed my baby . . . after surgery!" Some of the badges also address the popular beliefs of when to wean, such as "I breastfed my baby . . . after he could talk," "after she had teeth." They have versions of all of these with the word "chestfed" instead of "breastfed," and some badges refer to alternate ways of feeding a baby human milk (LLL USA 2015). These LLL badges are the ones that are most circulated in EN groups, although some people make their own badges or use images from other sites.

People who practice EN often mention being hesitant to share these as accomplishments on their main pages or with others, in part because of the negative feedback they have received in the past or are afraid they will receive. Another reason for not sharing more widely is that they are aware that this could be triggering or upsetting to friends and family who would have liked to nurse their children longer but were unable. Some of the badges from the LLL site do seem to be promoting the idea of always putting children's needs first and of nursing despite different health problems and discomfort. For many parents on EN sites, however, they provide some validation and celebration of the often unacknowledged work that was put into EN, even though many people who make this "choice" realize that the wider society would not think it was an accomplishment but instead as unnecessary, self-serving, or masochistic.

Mourning and Celebrating the End of the Nursing Journey

"You come to the end of an era, and they're not a little baby anymore and yeah, you always feel a little sad—a little bittersweet about those moments."

This is a quotation from Melissa, whose words I used to begin this chapter as well. People who practice EN often have mixed feelings about the end of the nursing relationship, even if it happens on their and/or the child's terms. In EN support groups, people often write about the end of the nursing relationship as complicated; like Melissa, they often use the word "bittersweet"; they might be relieved to be done, but they will also miss the close bond with their child (even though it of course does not end with weaning). In online groups, some people post or ask about the hormonal changes that might contribute to post-weaning depression. After weaning, EN parents often miss some of the perceived advantages of having nursing as a kind of "cure-all" for both minor and major emotional and physical trauma. Yet many people are also ready at a certain point to "have their body back," a common phrase in the EN community. When weaning is abrupt or when parents feel they and their child did not have agency in the weaning process, there is often a more intense sadness and frustration than if they were able to gently wean or if their child was able to self-wean.

Regardless of how weaning takes place, there are many ways that parents commemorate this journey both for themselves and for their children. One common practice that is discussed often in online spaces is having breast milk jewelry made for themselves and sometimes as a gift for their children. This is dried breast milk that is incorporated into decorative rings, necklaces, bracelets, and other jewelry. Although I did not ask questions about this jewelry in in-depth interviews, Paige mentioned wanting to do this, as she had saved a supply of frozen breast milk. Many parents in social media spaces also post photos of tattoos they have gotten to commemorate chest/breastfeeding, which include many colorful and either realistic or impressionistic images of the parent nursing a child or children or of something (often flowers or trees) that symbolizes the nursing experience for them.

For me, I think writing this book was my way of commemorating and remembering a time that was alternately difficult and wonderful but overall, to me as an anthropologist, endlessly interesting. In asking others about their experiences, I found so many stories that helped me further understand my own experiences and to see where they might diverge from that of other parents—not only because each child is different but because of the ways that people's backgrounds and circumstances play a part in the experience of EN.

8

"The Other Side of Milk"

Conclusion

An alternate title I considered for this book was "The Other Side of Milk," which was a phrase my son used to use to ask to switch "sides" (breasts), a common request for nursing children as milk supply might taper off and one breast is low on milk. This phrase also suggests different "sides" of the story of EN, including the experiences of people who practice EN and the opinions and practices of family, friends, medical and legal authorities, employers, and daycare operators. There is also the "side" related to local and national policy in relation to EN and weaning. In this chapter, I conclude the book by summarizing the findings of this research, in which I have attempted to document the perspectives of people practicing EN in the United States in the twenty-first century, and by discussing some considerations for the future of parent and child agency with EN. I also discuss some changes in the United States that have taken place both during and since concluding my research that have affected the experience of EN.

Facing Stigma, Seeking Support

Popular beliefs about an appropriate time for weaning, formed during the generations that passed when few children were nursed in the United States for more than a few months, if at all, and further shaped by cultural imaginaries about childhood and independence in a neoliberal capitalist society, were pervasive in interactions between my interlocutors and others. Since the 1970s, public and global health authorities have reintroduced chest/breastfeeding as something that is both accepted and expected, yet when nursing practices fall outside of certain parameters, parents and children may suffer the consequences of societal stigma. In this book, I focused on how people who nurse their child or children for two years or more experience stigma. In online posts in which an OP asks about the biggest and most difficult challenges with EN, many people will comment that it is dealing with other people and their stigmatizing attitudes. Some of these interactions were more consequential than others—for example, in the context of the medical encounter and in dealings with legal issues that affected family autonomy in decision-making related to when and how weaning would take place. Among my interviewees and in EN support groups, although people chest/breastfed their children for longer than is typical in the United States, some were compelled to wean earlier than they or their children might have wanted because of a number of circumstances; sometimes this was their own discomfort or another pregnancy, but often it was related to external pressures.

Many of the experiences I describe in this book reflect the challenges people have faced with EN stigma, but stories of my interlocutors also illustrate the kinds of support that make it possible to chest/breastfeed for as long as they did. "Support" can be complex and change over time; for example, a spouse or partner might support chest/breastfeeding in theory, but, like many people who practice EN, they do not always expect how transformative it can be to their lives for many years, impacting sleep spaces and patterns and sometimes affecting intimate relationships. Following the law (depending on the state) or by choice, an employer might support prolonged nursing by providing a space where a nursing parent can pump and store milk during the day, but that space might not be entirely private or sanitary. The research discussed in this book also highlights the degree to which having online support groups can be useful for EN parents, who might struggle to find support in other areas of their lives.

Online spaces can be particularly helpful in places where people do not have access to a La Leche group or other in-person support group and in cases where they feel they are the "only ones" in their circle of people they know who are "still" chest/breastfeeding. Private online groups on Facebook in which I was a participant observer provided validation of people's experiences; these were spaces where other people practicing EN offered both anecdotal and evidence-based information, often sharing links to peer-reviewed studies and AAP, LLL, and WHO websites. Members of these groups offered suggestions for addressing medical professionals or handling custody or visitation issues frequently. These were spaces where people also felt comfortable sharing stories about the experience of EN that might be perceived as "weird" or might be considered as perverse by people outside of the group. As one of my interviewees (Kim) noted, in discussing with her mom the irritation she felt surrounding twiddling behaviors (discussed in the last chapter) during nursing:

> My mom was like, I never even heard of that. I'm like, that's because you didn't have the internet [when her mom was nursing Kim and her siblings] and you didn't have access to other mothers. Get on an extended breastfeeding group. Thousands of members and, um, so breastfeeding comes up on there. Okay. There's definitely people have—twiddling is a thing. I was like, "no mom, lots of kids do this," you know.

Kim's comment reflects how online communities can provide a frame of reference and a sense of community. These groups can allow members to see that aspects of EN that might seem strange, even to those practicing it, are actually very common but perhaps hidden outside of these online communities.

In private Facebook groups, in over a decade of participating in these groups, I observed very few judgmental or negative comments about almost anything that people posted about, which is in part a testament to the site administrators, but the topic of gender identity and EN was an exception. In my observations, when the OPs identified themselves as nonbinary or transgender but AFAB, there would be a range of responses. Some comments were positive and mentioned that they or their partner were also nonbinary, and sometimes they would share some of the experiences related to that identity and how EN fit into that. Others might ask questions, mainly out of curiosity, particularly if something like "chestfeeding" was mentioned. However, there would also be a number of critical and transphobic comments; I witnessed some of these threads develop as people interacted in real time, often with comments related to the group being a safe space for people who identified as "women" only. Some commenters objected to or were put off by gender-neutral terms that they felt served to "erase" women. Looking back at these threads a few hours or days later, I would see that comments had been turned off, some of the comments had been removed, and the administrators had made statements about the comments breaking group non-discrimination rules, but the real-time development of some of these threads demonstrates that transphobia is rampant even within this community whose members are familiar with the effects of EN stigma. It was clear that some members either did not understand or did not tolerate the existence of people who did not identify as cisgender women in these spaces, which reflects both the growing visibility and the increasing hostility toward the transgender community in the United States. For some (at least as apparent in comments), gender nonconformity was perceived as a threat to more traditional concepts of "motherhood" as being exclusively for cisgender women. This double stigma that gender nonconforming parents who practice EN face is an important topic for future research, particularly as trans and nonbinary identities have been such a target of political rhetoric in the past few years.

Normalization and Destigmatization

Both interviewees and people in online support groups for EN expressed the desire for "normalizing" EN. Openness about EN can contribute to its normalization, which would certainly make life easier for people who choose to practice EN and child-led weaning. For lactating parents, however, being transparent about EN can feel risky. In writing this book, I hope that readers who may have had preconceived ideas about EN could come to see that nursing a child for two years or more is neither abnormal nor harmful. I also want to suggest that there can be many "normals" when it comes to infant and child feeding.

Imposing a single idea of what is most normal or that is for the "optimal" health of the child creates a new form of oppression. There is the danger of normalization causing problems for those who do not conform to a norm, particularly if there is a simplistic understanding of a singular norm for infant feeding. Townsend (2024), drawing on philosopher Michel Foucault's thoughts on the topic of societal norms set by powerful institutions, recently made this point as it relates to "homonormativity" at a university diversity office. She found that the wider acceptance of LGBTQ identities has resulted in normative expectations for identity, behavior, and appearance, so that those who fall outside of a norm are still subjects of stigma; for example, the new "normative" expectations for a trans person are that they conform to traditional gender roles in terms of clothing or hairstyle, but a person who identifies as nonbinary and does not clearly conform to the gender binary is likely to experience discrimination. Foucault made observations on the ways that "normalization" is about the standardization of practices, from educational "standards" to what is taught in medical school. He suggested that "the power of normalization imposes homogeneity" (1984: 196). The "Breast is Best" norm promoted by the global health community created pressure to conform and vilified those who could not, but it has done little to re-normalize EN in the United States, and in a sense, has generated increased stigma for those who practice EN with the backlash that has come from this campaign. "Fed is Best" is one alternative that approaches the idea of "many normals" for infant and child feeding (The Fed is Best Foundation 2020); this is the concept of providing support for many forms of feeding a child, including chest/breastfeeding from the body, bottle feeding of pumped milk, bottle feeding with formula, or a combination, though the phrase "fed is best" is contested by some who feel that the overly simplistic nature of this phrase could have negative health consequences for infants.

EN and child-led weaning would theoretically be seen as more normal (or at least less stigmatized) if there were policies in place at the national level that could facilitate more people being able to make choices about chest/breastfeeding and weaning practices. In online groups and among my interviewees, flexible work policies and family leave have helped people who wanted to practice EN and child-led weaning, but policy alone does not destigmatize this practice, however. Norway, for example, has a generous paid parental leave policy, and chest/breastfeeding is strongly encouraged and supported at the national level, but Therese Andrews' (2022) found that stigma persists for lactating parents on both ends of a spectrum of nursing duration. Those who have difficulties establishing or would prefer not to nurse their children feel vilified and people who continue to nurse their children for "too long" (as early as eighteen months) feel judged; both are made to feel as if they are harming their children. The taboo against EN is understood to keep "the child from being used by his/her mother for the mother's own benefits and protects the child's psychological or emotional development from being jeopardized" (Andrews 2022: 67–8). I mention this study in Norway not to suggest that generous parental leave policies are not helpful to families but rather that they have not resulted in EN being seen as normal. These policies can certainly make it easier for EN to take place. In the United States, the polar opposite extreme of limited to no paid parental leave and limited support for childcare complicates child rearing and feeding for the majority of families, which leads to threats to the short and long-term health of infants and children. Among my interviewees who practiced EN, some mentioned how the flexibility of their work situations (e.g., having breaks to pump milk or having a daycare on site at the workplace or living in states where employers were mandated to provide breaks for pumping milk) made it possible for them to nurse their child or children for two years or more.

People who practice EN play different roles in attempting to normalize this practice, or at least in attempting to show others that it is not "out of place." Some are very vocal and open about EN while others choose to conceal or not disclose the fact that they are nursing. The latter approach is about wanting to circumvent expected stigma, which many had already experienced in earlier phases of nursing their children. Crystal, who was from a state in the Midwest, said that she had stopped telling both friends and family that she was still nursing:

> I'm not necessarily ashamed, but people in my area and circle of friends just do not make it easy to talk about [it], or then have their own ideas on what it looks like for them, and it can be challenging to get a point across.

Caitlyn talked about how she never nursed in front of her father because she knew he "was really uncomfortable with any bodily function. And I think he would be really embarrassed; I was trying to save him embarrassment," although she also questioned her own decision and asked whether it was worthwhile to "save" others in this way. As noted in the last chapter, though, she was open about the fact that she was nursing her infant when she was teaching middle school students, and this openness could have an impact on the next generation. With EN, however, it was common for parents to disclose the fact that they were still nursing to as few people as possible in order to avoid the hassle of explaining it or to avoid stigma. They or their children were sometimes compelled to disclose this information for medical reasons or in some legal contexts, but otherwise, many EN parents were more private about EN as their children got older. This nondisclosure is understandable but can also contribute to EN continuing to seem like a practice that is strange and "out of place" in the contemporary United States.

EN as Harm Reduction in Global Health?

The compounding effects of climate change, conflict, migration, and global inequality contribute to increasingly precarious situations for children's health worldwide. Chary et al. have suggested that the WHO pushes breastfeeding for two years or more as a way to address infant malnutrition globally in lieu of attempting to "implement various infrastructural improvement and food security programs that would also effectively address the issue of maternal-child health" (2011: 180). For example, Mehta et al. called EN "an inexpensive public health service to developing countries" (2017: 143), as it allows for greater birth spacing and lowers child mortality. These issues could also, or instead, be addressed through better sanitation and healthcare services in rural areas and access to birth control and family planning. However, Chary et al. noted that promoting EN is more appealing to public and global health policymakers since investments of the magnitude that would decrease wealth disparities and improve health outcomes for children would require massive political will, "whereas exclusive breastfeeding does not" (2011: 180). In this sense, chest/breastfeeding and EN become neoliberal solutions (in terms of less investment being required from governments) and represent a strategy of pharmaceuticalization (making breast milk into medicine) that draws on the unpaid labor of women and other lactating parents. Suggesting chest/breastfeeding and EN as solutions to global health issues does acknowledge the value of these practices in theory, but there is rarely concomitant support or remuneration for families to recognize its value. In an article in *The Atlantic* that is critical of the breastfeeding imperative that has come to be pushed on women, Rosin has suggested that

> by insisting that milk is some kind of vaccine, they make it less likely that we'll experience nursing primarily as a loving maternal act—"pleasant and relaxing," in the words of *Our Bodies, Ourselves*—and more likely that we'll view it as, well, dispensing medicine. (2009: 68)

As noted in the previous chapter, some of my interlocutors did see their breast milk in this utilitarian way, and some felt an obligation to nurse as long as they could for the long-term health and well-being of their children (and themselves). Often, they talked about this in positive ways, though, giving examples of how nursing their child served to soothe physical or emotional pain or how they felt they were able to give extra protection to their children during the pandemic by passing on antibodies from the Covid vaccine.

EN, Feminism, Lactivism, and Parenting Agency

Some scholars and individuals have suggested that EN and other practices associated with an attachment or intensive parenting model are anti-feminist in that they require an inordinate output of time and unpaid labor from women and people of other marginalized identities who are practicing EN. Cappellini et al. noted that in Europe and the United States, the

> intensification of motherhood . . . requires mothers not only to put their child's needs before their own in every respect, but to be able to display this to others through their everyday practices. (2019: 471)

The parents I interviewed were aware of these pressures of "good motherhood/parenting," but they felt that chest/breastfeeding was the best choice for their child, given the information with which they were familiar. However, EN was more of an "accidental" phenomenon that happened after chest/breastfeeding was well-established; some of my interlocutors saw EN and child-led weaning as more laid-back parenting options that would have been much easier if family, medical, societal, and other pressures to wean were not so strong. After their children had weaned, some parents in interviews and EN online groups lamented the loss of tools that they had for soothing a child's emotions or helping their child fall asleep and missed the closeness they experienced with their child during this time. Others did talk or write about the intensity and time commitment of the EN experience and sometimes exerted self-pressure to continue nursing, sometimes pushing past their own discomfort and past external pressures to wean, for what they perceived as their children's benefit—or more often because parental attempts to wean an older child required more intensive labor and stress than child-led weaning. However, in these groups, when someone posted that they were still nursing "only for the child's sake," despite being uncomfortable or wishing the nursing relationship to end, comments generally favored encouraging people to prioritize their own health and well-being and offered advice for gentle weaning.

My interviewees did not identify as "lactivists" (which is a question I asked them, in terms of promoting chest/breastfeeding and EN as optimal parenting). In contrast, many were hesitant to talk to family, friends, and others about their choices, or they became hesitant after experiencing stigma. However, a few of my interview participants had become lactation consultants or LLL leaders after the experience of practicing EN themselves, because they wanted to make this experience easier for others. In my own experience, I construed my choice to practice child-led weaning as a human right, though there are no formal legal protections in the United States for parents/children who make this choice. I have felt compelled to write this book and advocate for those who encounter stigmatizing attitudes or policies that limit their agency. I would advocate for the conditions that would make it practical and feasible to practice EN; I also think it is important as an anthropologist to point out that EN was common throughout much of human prehistory and cross-culturally, that it is safe (with no evidence-based research showing otherwise), and that the idea of EN as "abnormal" is one that is a product of a confluence of historical and cultural factors.

Shifting Milkscapes in the United States and Globally

All ethnographic research is representative of the particular time and place in which it is conducted; by the time an ethnographic study gets published, much may have already changed. The fact that it has taken me over a decade to complete my research and publish this book has given me a longitudinal perspective on other people's experiences with EN during some drastic societal changes, including changes to the digital and social media landscape and the effects of the Covid-19 pandemic on parenting and work. I used "milkscapes" in the title of this section, casually drawing on Arjun Appadurai's delineation of different "scapes" (e.g., mediascapes, technoscapes) that help us understand "the dimensions of global cultural flows" which "point to the fluid, irregular shapes of these landscapes" (2005: 33); this seems like an apt metaphor for breast milk and how child feeding and weaning practices fit into local and global changes.

I started thinking about doing this research when my son was still dependent on nursing to fall asleep, and as I write this, he is getting ready to start college. In the final stages of the research and writing of this book, I started to feel like it had been too long since I stopped being a nursing parent to be able to relate to a younger generation of EN parents. Sam, one of my interviewees, expressed similar feelings in discussing her work as a lactation consultant:

> I do feel that there is a time limit placed on me to continue doing work for moms. So I'm about to wean this child [her second], and that makes me not a breastfeeding mom anymore. The authority that I have as a person who is currently lactating when I walk in to see a [lactating parent] is very, very different than if I said, "Oh, I haven't breastfed in five years." And some people want that grandmotherly relationship, and they'll hire these lactation professionals who are in their fifties or sixties, but some people want that sisterly peer relationship, and I see that I'm going to lose that . . . One of the women that I shadowed in lactation [consulting] had been working in rotation for 43 years. And some of the things that I learned from her are completely and utterly irrelevant or we have science to show that [things have changed]. And she's a genius.

Sam talked about how it was not only about personal distance from chest/breastfeeding but also cultural changes creating a generational gap between herself and her clients:

> The other thing that I see of technology is changing. Technology is changing the way we breastfeed. My mother-in-law talks about how she would read books and watch TV while she breastfeeds; now people are on their phones. But there's an

interaction on social media on message boards that's quiet while you're nursing. ... So it's changing the way we breastfeed and, a generation, ten years from now, the way I breastfed my kids will not be the way my clients are breastfeeding their children. Because it's changing so rapidly, I feel like I'm going to move out of the one-on-one consulting and counseling and into public policy development for research, because I'm going to expire. I'm going to be old for the field.

I was sometimes frustrated by not being able to get this book completed more quickly. At the same time, ethnographic research does not have to involve a completely overlapping or shared identity with participants. Over the years, when I would mention my research to someone who was practicing or had practiced EN, they would say that it was important to tell these stories, and I felt a strong obligation to complete this work.

Some of my interviewees were able to reflect on changes from the time they had their first child (around the same time that my son was born) and their experience with a second child in terms of hospital experiences and lactation support. In Chapter 3, I included Melissa's story of a 2007 hospital experience that could have easily derailed her attempts to breastfeed in the first place and a contrasting, more supportive hospital birth experience in 2018. Paige also talked about the "very different experience" she had with two children, born ten years apart, speculating that it could be because "times change" but also the different locations (though both of her children were born in rural counties in the US Southeast). While she had very little support for nursing her first child, she said that with her second, "They had a color code on [her son's] name tag that was on his bassinet, and it basically meant, like, do not give him a bottle if it had that sticker." Their contrasting experiences could reflect an overall increase in support for chest/breastfeeding in recent years, with a good model for ways to establish and maintain the nursing relationship, but these practices have not been implemented everywhere and may depend on insurance coverage or funding for government-sponsored programs in the future.

The span of time that this research has covered has been one during which there have been some significant shifts in culture, technology, healthcare, and politics. Over the past decade, I have also witnessed and participated in the growth in online communities and discussions about EN, and I have seen an increase in the need in these communities for knowledge that can be presented as informed when members interact with others who attempt to undermine their parenting decisions. Through the conclusion of my formal research in 2024 and as I write this in 2025, I continue to see frequent posts in online support groups about all of the issues I covered in this book, including stigmatizing attitudes about EN experienced in a variety of settings but also examples of ways that others did offer support, which was most freely given if another person had personal experience with or exposure to EN.

Since formally beginning this project in 2012, new online platforms and formats for sharing information and digital storytelling have emerged, including "stories" (temporary photos or videos that are highlighted on a social media account, often just for twenty-four hours), reels (videos you create that are permanently in your feed), and live sessions on Instagram, YouTube, Facebook, and TikTok. There is also no guarantee that these platforms will persist. In early 2025, for example, there were discussions of TikTok vanishing for users in the United States because of Congressional concerns about user data being accessed by the Chinese government; if access to TikTok continues, new privacy concerns could emerge with a takeover by US-based CEOs politically aligned with groups that might threaten users' privacy and safety. Out of concerns about Meta's lack of protection against hate speech and its own forms of censorious action, private groups in which there are fears about legal issues are migrating rapidly to other platforms and deleting entire support groups. Other ethnographers have experienced these shifts, which are prompted by many intersecting forces. David Nemer's (2022) work in favela communities in Brazil, initially with a focus on LAN (Local Area Network) houses where people could go to access the internet, demonstrates the rapidity of change; as more people got their own smartphones, these LAN houses became less used and less common. He also documented the migration of Brazilians from the platforms Orkut to Facebook to WhatsApp. Linguistic anthropologist Kendra Calhoun's early research (2016, 2019) took place on Vine, a platform that was shut down in 2017, and she has since shifted some of her work to focus on TikTok. As these spaces shift though, their earlier research remains relevant; the rapid shift in the digital landscape highlights how important it is to do research in these spaces to both document historical uses of the internet and to understand the present moment. On a podcast ("That Anthro Podcast"), Calhoun mentions the "lingering influence of Vine, particularly the style of videos that people post on social media" (interview by Campbell 2022: Online). However, the shutdown or banning of certain platforms can result in the loss of access to information that serves as a cultural archive. Working in digital spaces requires ethnographers to be particularly flexible, though arguably this is true of all ethnography in a rapidly changing world.

The Covid-19 pandemic also occurred during my window of research, and I had a chance to see some of its mixed effects on people who were practicing EN. There were some negative effects on chest/breastfeeding initiation for newer parents, which may have long-term consequences; for example, DeYoung and Mangum (2021) noted that Covid precautions sometimes resulted in new parents being separated from their infants if they tested positive for Covid, and people had more limited access to in-person medical care or access to lactation consultants. There were also interesting positive developments that came out of the pandemic for some parents. During the stricter quarantine phase of the pandemic, a few parents I interviewed described enjoying a time that was free from judgment of others if they were able to primarily stay at home and perhaps have less contact with relatives or others who might have something negative to say about their parenting decisions. Work from home offers greater freedom in parenting choices and flexibility to nurse on demand, but it also resutls in an increased burden on working parents who are primary caregivers.

As Covid numbers dropped and vaccines and boosters were more accessible, many employers continue to allow for more flexibility with work schedules in jobs where remote work is possible and even more practical than in-person work. For those who have this option for work in the future, the opportunity to practice EN and child-led weaning might be opening up to more people. For many working-class parents whose jobs have not been converted to even a partially virtual option, nothing changed in terms of the limited options for establishing long-term chest/breastfeeding relationships through extended time at home. For parents/caregivers who do have the privilege to work part-time or full-time from their homes, when this work is coupled with childcare, parents/caregivers experience a double burden. There has also been (in 2025) a trend toward "return to work," following mandates at the federal level that are impacting other institutions, especially those that receive some support from the federal government.

Recent political upheaval in the United States may prove to significantly affect families and the autonomy and agency of chest/breastfeeding parents. As I write this (in 2025), many of the directives laid out in Project 2025 are being introduced through legislation and executive orders under the current presidential administration. Though immigrant detention and deportation were existing practices that negatively affected nursing parents, recent reports of parents being separated or deported separately from their nursing children have been making it to the news (Walters 2025), as in the recent case of a Cuban woman who was not given the option of taking her 17-month-old daughter (who was still nursing) with her when she was deported in May 2025. The ratcheting up of legislation and rhetoric associated with the LGBTQIA+ community, with a particular emphasis on the trans community, could have a long-lasting impact on trans people's agency in parenting decisions. So far it is unclear if additional steps will be made to mandate paid leave for parents, despite an emphasis in Project 2025 on family and "traditional" values. In this plan, it is suggested that there be fewer regulations for the production and sale of formula (The Heritage Foundation 2024: 301). The justification for loosening these regulations was the formula shortage that took place "during the Biden Administration," although the reasons for this shortage were more complicated, including the Covid-19 pandemic and the general lack of support for nursing parents throughout the country. Asiodou (2022: 341) noted that though the shortage was not a new issue, its severity during the pandemic "devolved into a breast-feeding-versus-formula-feeding battle," rather than focusing on the problems with policies "that prioritize capitalistic goals and corporate profits over human milk feeding and the health and wellbeing of birthing and lactating parents." The proposed loosening of regulations for formula production could potentially increase the supply but also increase the risk of contamination (and the need for mass recall, leading to more shortages); for parents who have the opportunities to nurse their children longer, they might feel compelled to do so, while others who are not able to will face greater risks to their children's health through potentially substandard formula.

Final Thoughts

My intention in doing this research and writing this book has never been to suggest that everyone *should* nurse their children for two years or more or until they self-wean. Although there can be physiological and emotional benefits to EN for those who practice it and for their children, given wider societal issues and external pressures, the stressors associated with EN often outweigh these benefits. Instead, my purpose was to tell the stories of people (including my own) who have practiced EN in the United States in these first decades of the twenty-first century to both describe different aspects of EN and to highlight some of the ways that this experience was made either easier through support systems online or in person or unnecessarily difficult by those for whom EN was seen as an abnormal or harmful parenting practice. This view of EN as harmful, based on lack of exposure to chest/breastfeeding in general and especially lack of knowledge of "what it looks like" and what it means to nurse a child who can walk and talk, often has real implications in social, healthcare, and legal settings.

It is my hope that in writing and talking about this research, people who practice EN may feel seen and perhaps be able to utilize this text to demonstrate to others that their choice to continue nursing beyond what is often considered "normal" in the United States is not bad parenting. I also hope that this book could play even a small part in helping people, especially those in positions in which they have power and authority over others' bodies and parenting choices, to see EN as one practice among many "normals" for child feeding/weaning. I believe attitudes can change, often with simple exposure to different ideas and practices; the story I described in the introduction, about sharing information with one of my physicians who regularly made jokes about it being "time to wean" if a child can ask for a sandwich with "milk on the side," is one example of how quickly ideas can shift. For many people who practice EN, the authority they have to speak to these issues is questioned, so further academic research on this topic can be useful.

Appendix A
In-depth Interview Questions

The following questions were approved by Georgia State University's Institutional Review Board. I had two separate IRB applications (H13343; H190855) as one expired before I was able to do a continuing review. These are the most recently approved (in 2022) questions for in-depth interviews.

Background information

Can you tell me your age?

How do you identify in terms of ethnicity, race, and/or family background?

Can you give me some information about your background? (Where did you grow up? When did you move to Atlanta?)

What's your educational background?

Do you work currently? If so, what positions?

Are you currently married or do you have a partner you live with?

How many children do you have? What are their ages?

Decisions about Breastfeeding

What were some of the reasons why you chose to breastfeed in the first place?

Does extended breastfeeding fit in with a particular parenting style you follow?

Did you have any problems getting started with one or more of your children?

If you work or have worked outside the home, what challenges or positive experiences have you had in continuing breastfeeding?

Did you also use a pump at some point? Would your child drink from a bottle?

Discuss any physical problems that you had with breastfeeding in the first weeks or months.

Did you intend to breastfeed for more than two years? If not, how long did you think you would breastfeed? What factors played a part in breastfeeding longer than you thought you might?

If you planned to breastfeed for a longer time, what were some of the reasons?

Were you breastfed as a child?

What role do you feel your child has/had in extended breastfeeding?

When breastfeeding ended (if it has), do you feel it was child-led? Did you change your behaviors at all in order to encourage the weaning process?

Did/does your child nurse to fall asleep?

Do you/have you practiced co-sleeping?

Can you discuss how breastfeeding changed in terms of timing and frequency over the years of your child's life (from infancy to the present or to when breastfeeding ceased)?

Once your child was able to talk, how did that change the experience of breastfeeding? What were some other developmental changes that made this experience different?

What changes in your life during this time made breastfeeding different?

Stigma and Support

Did you have support from your family in your decisions about breastfeeding?

Are you/have you been supported by your partner/spouse? Have you ever had disagreements with your partner about extended breastfeeding?

Have you breastfed an older child (about two years old or older) in a public setting? Why or why not?

If not, can you think of some things that would make it more comfortable for you to breastfeed in public?

Have you experienced discrimination or negative behaviors from others in public settings? If so, can you give some examples?

Talking about Breastfeeding

Do you discuss the fact that your child is being/was breastfed with any friends? With colleagues at work? With family members? What factors are involved in your decision to tell some people but not others?

If you don't let others know, how do you conceal this information?

Do you consider yourself an activist or lactivist?

What do you think the benefits of extended breastfeeding were to you and your child? Any drawbacks?

Appendix B
Participant Profiles

In-Depth Interview Participant Demographic Profiles

Ages for participants and children reflect the time of interview; all were married or partnered or had at one point been married or partnered with cisgender men. The racial identities are in quotation marks because I asked people to self-identify, so these are the answers they provided in the interview.

2017 Interviews

Ashley (interview at her house): age twenty-nine; "white"; from the Southeast, moved later to a state in the Southwest; graduate student in social science; two kids at the time of interview; recently divorced at the time of the in-depth interview.

Stephanie (interview in person in my campus office): age thirty-five; "white"; from the Southeast; public health background, graduate degree; one child, two years old, not yet weaned; married.

Sam (interview in person, coffee shop): thirty-five; background/identity; "It's always complicated. I identify as white, I also identify as Jewish, I don't identify my sexuality. I am married to a man who identifies as a cishet male"; from the Southeast; two kids, aged seven and three; currently nursing the three-year-old; degrees in fine arts and creative writing; currently working as a lactation counselor and pediatric nutritionist.

Anne (interview at a coffee shop): thirty-nine; "Caucasian/white/European"; grew up in the Southeast, went to college on the West Coast; nursing school in the Southeast; currently an oncology nurse; two children; nursed her six-year-old for about four and a half years and was still nursing her three-year-old; practiced tandem nursing for a while; married.

Richa (interview at a restaurant): thirty-nine; "Asian/Indian American"; born and grew up in a Mid-Atlantic state; now lives in the Southeast; graduate degree; currently works in public health; two children (age eight and ten) both weaned at the time of interview; she nursed her youngest for a little less than two years and her oldest for over three years; married.

Interviews 2022–4

Amy (virtual interview): forty-one; "white"; living in the Midwest; two children, ages seven and three who practiced EN with both—her first child for two and a half years before the child self-weaned; second child is still nursing at three; attorney and La Leche leader; married.

Deanna (virtual interview): forty-two; "multiracial" (mom is white, dad is Black/African-American); born and spent some time in the Midwest as a child; has resided in the Southeast for over two decades; social science undergraduate degree; one child nursed until age three, weaned recently; working as contracts manager in public health; divorced from her child's father and, at the time of interview, partnered with a man who also has a child.

Caitlyn (virtual interview): age thirty-six; "white/European descent"; grew up and lives in the Southeast; one child who just turned five and stopped nursing at three and a half; she was thirty-four weeks pregnant with her second child at the time of interview; social science background with a graduate degree in education; taught middle school for two years, worked for a while as a teacher after this child was born, but then left this position and got her IBCLC Certification; married.

Melissa (virtual interview): age forty-seven; "white"; grew up in the Southeast, has lived in the Northeast, currently in the Southeast; practiced EN with four children; at the time of the interview, her children are between the ages of four and fifteen; four-year-old was still nursing; tandem nursed during the pandemic;

works in insurance disability claims; divorced and remarried, with children from both marriages.

Gabby (virtual interview): age twenty-eight; "Black and Mexican American" (mom is from Mexico, father is African American); born in the Midwest and still lives there; works as a medical assistant; one child, age two and a half; married.

Kim (virtual interview): age forty-six; "white/Caucasian"; from a Mid Atlantic state originally, now living in the Southeast; degree in engineering and worked in this field for a while but currently a stay-at-home mom; one child who is three and a half and still nursing; married.

Nia (virtual interview): age twenty-eight, "Black/African American"; middle/lower middle class; originally from a Western state, has lived in the Southeast for several years; graduate degree in social science and seeking another graduate degree in nurse midwifery; one child breastfed for two years; worked as a doula and got her IBCLC; married.

Michelle (virtual interview): age forty-seven, "white"; grew up and living in the Northeast; middle/upper middle class; MD degree; physician, professor, and researcher; child was three years old, weaned at about two and a half; married.

Paige (virtual interview); age twenty-nine, "white," middle class/lower middle class background; from the Southeast; undergraduate and graduate degree in a social science; children are eleven and three; practiced EN with her second child; married.

Below are pseudonyms I use in the book for other participants whose stories I used in the book and with whom I was in touch through social media interactions/messaging. I gained their consent to use paraphrased versions of stories they discussed with me through PM or in social media posts but did not conduct formal interviews with them and so I have limited information about their identities:

Jenny, "white," dental health professional, from the Southeast; two children.

Allison, "white," from the Northeast; two children.

Crystal, "white," from the Midwest, one child.

Meg, "white," from the Midwest, nursed one child for over three years.

Jocelyn, "Asian/Filipina American," born in the Philippines, living in the Midwest; one child, nursed beyond age four.

Shelby, "white," from the Southwest; one child, nursed until her child turned four.

Appendix C
Court Letter for Parents Practicing EN

I am writing to provide an academic perspective on breastfeeding practices. I am a medical anthropologist in the Department of Anthropology at Georgia State University, and I am currently doing research on women's experiences of "extended breastfeeding" and stigma in the United States. "Extended" is a relative term because it is difficult to pinpoint an age where it is "natural" for humans to wean, though if we look to our close primate relatives, the great apes, which have life spans comparable to humans, nurse their offspring for six years or more. Both the World Health Organization's and the American Academy of Pediatrics' recommendation for breastfeeding is two years or beyond. The data are accumulating on the long-term benefits of extended breastfeeding—aside from benefits in terms of nutrition and the passing on of antibodies from mother to child (which continues as long as children continue to breastfeed, contrary to popular belief) for children, extended breastfeeding can lead to reduced risk of obesity and a lowered incidence of non-communicable diseases in children.

Breastfeeding in general became less practiced globally with the introduction of formula feeding, but some of the short- and long-term negative consequences of formula have prompted national and global health organizations to push more strongly for women to breastfeed. Breastfeeding toddlers and young children was fairly commonplace in past generations in the United States and was done publicly with no social repercussions. However, the fact that formula feeding was the norm for a few decades of US history means that breastfeeding itself came to seem strange or out of place. In addition, many women are unable to breastfeed beyond a few weeks because they do not have adequate support to initiate lactation or because they do not have a flexible work schedule or a place to breastfeed or pump their milk. In the United States and much of the Western world today, most people are unaccustomed to seeing women breastfeeding at all and thus are shocked by seeing or hearing about toddlers or young children nursing. Though still in the minority, the number of women who are able to practice "child-led weaning," in which they breastfeed until children are ready to stop, is growing in the United States, with tens of thousands of people participating in online support groups related to extended breastfeeding and child-led weaning.

In practice, there is a wide range of weaning ages among people cross-culturally—from a few days to seven or more years. There are no documented psychological issues with extending breastfeeding until the child and/or mother feels ready to wean, and having interviewed many women who breastfed for several years, it is clear that no parents did this to satisfy their personal needs; they chose to continue the nursing relationship because they believed it was the best thing for the child (emotionally and nutritionally) and/or because their children continued to need to nurse.

During times of family stress, such as divorce, breastfeeding can provide a source of immense comfort to children. On the contrary, abrupt weaning during this time can be extremely stressful. Breastfeeding does not have to result in the exclusion of the other parent from children's lives. All parents and caretakers can be active in children's lives through close contact, affection, and spending time with children. I think in situations of separation and divorce, both parents should prioritize the interests and mental health of the children—nursing children who are not accustomed to overnight separation from their mothers, particularly for several days in a row on repeated occasions, will most likely experience a significant amount of stress and anxiety. There can be a commitment on the part of both parents to make sure the children will be able to adapt to the custody arrangement in their own time.

It is noteworthy that there is a history of fathers attempting to use breastfeeding as a means to demonstrate a mother's lack of fitness in custody hearings, even when they had previously been supportive of extended breastfeeding and child-led weaning (Baldwin 2001). However, fathers who are patient and understand and appreciate their children's needs will be able to have a strong and healthy relationship with their children throughout their children's lives. It is my professional opinion that mothers should be allowed to continue breastfeeding as long as it works for both her and her children. Overnight visits away from the nursing parent are not conducive to maintaining breastfeeding, particularly in the first few years of a child's life. Quality time spent with the father is still possible through day visits, which are a great way for fathers to bond with their child.

Please feel free to contact me if you have any questions or concerns or would like more academic evidence related to extended breastfeeding. Thank you.

Sincerely,
Cassandra White

Notes

Chapter 1

1 The topic of breast cancer screening for nursing parents is addressed in Chapter 5.
2 "Child-led weaning" is distinct from the parenting strategy known as "baby-led weaning" (Rapley and Murkett 2008), which is an infant feeding strategy in which a wide variety of solid foods (as opposed to commercial baby foods), including any foods that adults would be eating, are introduced during the first year of life, with the idea children will develop a broader palate and better socialization skills. The use of "weaning" in this term has to do with the idea that introducing solid foods is part of the transition to weaning from breast milk, but theoretically people can practice both child-led weaning from breast milk and baby-led weaning as a feeding strategy.
3 In retrospect, I could have/wish I had collected more detailed demographic information about these participants as a part of the research process, but I initially thought I would mainly be paraphrasing their comments from social media posts and comments. In some cases, through messaging, I did have a chance to learn a lot about these participant's lives and situations, particularly in relation to the topic of their original post.

Chapter 2

1 "Neoliberal" refers to economies in which markets (buying and selling of goods, commodities, products, ideas—anything that can be bought or sold) operate with relative freedom from government regulations.
2 "Interlocutor" is a term used by cultural and linguistic anthropologists to refer to research participants; they might be interviewees or people with whom we interact as part of participant observation. "Interlocutor" replaces the term "informant," one that many anthropologists used in the past, but the negative connotations of "informant" (e.g., as someone who spies on or provides secret information about others) have come to be understood as problematic.
3 There have been some attempts to calculate the "cost" of chest/breastfeeding versus formula feeding. The idea of chest/breastfeeding as a "free" source of food for a child does not take into account the time and possible lost wages that this form of feeding might entail. A recent study by Mahoney et al. (2023), suggests

that nursing a child can be more costly than formula feeding in calculations they performed that included the "hidden costs" of things like lost wages, additional caloric needs for the lactating parent, and long-term effects, like the cost of slower job progression because of caregiving responsibilities. They noted that based on these calculations, these effects would be more felt by lower-income families who have less job flexibility, though the point of the study was also to suggest ways that chest/breastfeeding parents could be more supported and that this practice could become less costly to families. However, Bartick et al. (2017) also used a modeling framework to estimate the high costs of "suboptimal breastfeeding" (with optimal defined as six months of exclusive nursing) in the United States, using existing studies related to relative benefits of nursing for lactating parents and children, focusing on the hypothetical medical costs that could arise from disease and mortality outcomes for both lactating parents and children that are associated with suboptimal nursing. In their model, the costs of "suboptimal breastfeeding" were higher for women's long-term health than for infant health.

Chapter 3

1 In contemporary anthropology, we no longer use the term "primitive" to refer to any society, because "primitive" has the negative connotations of suggesting a society that is less advanced or inferior to others. Anthropologists used this term in the past to describe non-industrialized societies or societies whose economies were based on foraging (hunting, gathering, fishing) and/or horticulture (small-scale agriculture). In Margaret Mead's research, she attempted to describe aspects of Samoan culture (e.g., more openness regarding sex, gender, sexuality, and death and less of a generation gap than in the United States) that she considered a model that led to less angst and conflict than was typical of US adolescence at the time (Mead 2001, original 1928).
2 Although the AAP updated its official stance on weaning since Dettwyler wrote this, many pediatricians still push for earlier weaning than many EN parents are comfortable with, as will be discussed in Chapter 5.

Chapter 4

1 I include "Jewish" here because this is part of how she self-identified in a question about her racial and ethnic identity.
2 In Chapter 5, I go into more detail about dental care, caries, and chest/breastfeeding.

Chapter 5

1. See also White (2024) for a more extensive discussion of Deanna's experience.
2. See Carnino et al. for details on different oral ties, all of which are the result of "unusually" short or thickened tissue connecting the underside of the tongue (tongue/lingual tie), the upper lip (lip/labial tie), or cheek (cheek/buccal tie) to other parts of the mouth, which can affect the establishment of nursing in the first place but can also lead to the "inability to clean the oral cavity" (2023: 1 of 6).
3. WIC is the "Special Supplemental Nutrition Program for Women, Infants, and Children," a US federally funded program that provides nutritional support (in the form of food and formula, for example) and counseling for lower-income people who are pregnant, nursing a child, formula-feeding a child, or have a young child in need of additional food supplements. They also provide nutritional counseling and lactation support (USDA 2024).

Chapter 7

1. Comments are paraphrased from a public social media page.

References

Adler, Christina J., Keith Dobney, Laura S. Weyrich, John Kaidonis, Alan W. Walker, Wolfgang Haak, Corey J. A. Bradshaw, Grant Townsend Arkadiusz Sołtysiak, Kurt Alt, Julian Parkhill, and Alan Cooper (2013), "Sequencing Ancient Calcified Dental Plaque Shows Changes in Oral Microbiota with Dietary Shifts of the Neolithic and Industrial Revolutions," *Nature Genetics*, 45(4): 450–5.

Albadran, Maysara M. (2013), "Effect of Breastfeeding during Pregnancy on the Occurrence of Miscarriage and Preterm Labour," *Iraqi Journal of Medical Sciences*, 11(3): 285–98.

Alvarado, Gabriela (2025), "How Workplaces Should Design Lactation Rooms: A Wishlist Informed by Clinical Practice, Maternal Health Research, and Personal Experience as a Breastfeeding Mom," *Breastfeeding Medicine*, 20(2): 88–90.

AAP (2021), "Breastfeeding Overview," Available online: https://www.aap.org/en/patient-care/breastfeeding/breastfeeding-overview/ (accessed March 30, 2024).

AAP (2024), "Safe Sleep," Available online: https://www.aap.org/en/patient-care/safe-sleep/ (accessed August 1, 2024).

Anderson, Benedict (2006), *Imagined Communities: Reflections on the Origin and Spread of Nationalism*, New York: Verso Books.

Andrews, Therese (2022), "Modern Taboos and Moral Regulations: Mother's Milk in the Symbolic Order," *Sociology*, 56(1): 55–71.

Appadurai, Arjun (2005), *Modernity at Large: Cultural Dimensions of Globalization*, Minneapolis/London: University of Minnesota Press.

Ashe, Leah M. (2021), "From Iatrogenic Harm to Iatrogenic Violence: Corruption and the End of Medicine," *Anthropology & Medicine*, 28(2): 255–75.

Asiodou, Ifeyinwa V. (2022), "Infant Formula Shortage: This Should Not Be Our Reality," *The Journal of Perinatal and Neonatal Nursing*, 36(4): 340–3.

Baldwin, Elizabeth (2001), "Extended Breastfeeding and the Law," *Breastfeeding Abstracts*, 20(3): 19–20.

Bartick, Melissa C., Eleanor Bimla Schwarz, Brittany D. Green, Briana J. Jegier, Arnold G. Reinhold, Tarah T. Colaizy, Debra L. Bogen, Andrew J. Schaefer, and Alison M. Stuebe (2017), "Suboptimal Breastfeeding in the United States: Maternal and Pediatric Health Outcomes and Costs," *Maternal & Child Nutrition*, 13(1): e12366.

Bartick, Melissa, Elizabeth K. Stehel, Sarah L. Calhoun, Lori Feldman-Winter, Deena Zimmerman, Lawrence Noble, Casey Rosen-Carole, Laura R. Kair, and Academy of Breastfeeding Medicine (2021), "Academy of Breastfeeding Medicine Position

Statement and Guideline: Infant Feeding and Lactation-related Language and Gender," *Breastfeeding Medicine*, 16(8): 587–90.

Baynham, Justin T. L., M. Allison Moorman, Catherine Donnellan, Vicky Cevallos, and Jeremy D. Keenan (2013), "Antibacterial Effect of Human Milk for Common Causes of Paediatric Conjunctivitis," *British Journal of Ophthalmology*, 97(3): 377–9.

Bentley, Amy (2006), "Booming Baby Food: Infant Food and Feeding in Post-World War II America," *Michigan Historical Review*, 32(2): 63–87.

Bertoia, Carl, and Janice Drakich (1993), "The Fathers' Rights Movement: Contradictions in Rhetoric and Practice," *Journal of Family Issues*, 14(4): 592–615.

Bertollo, Leandro Pedro Goloni, Liliana Alice da Silva Campos, Thaiane Almeida Suzuki, Meily Soares Chao, Vanessa Cunha dos Santos, Ana Paula Andreotti Amorim, and Ana Claudia Camargo Gonçalves Germani (2024), "Lactation Induction for Transgender Women and Transfeminine People in Health Care: A Scoping Review," *Ciência & Saúde Coletiva*, 29: e18232023.

Bird-David, Nurit (2008), "Feeding Nayaka Children and English Readers: A Bifocal Ethnography of Parental Feeding in 'The Giving Environment,'" *Anthropological Quarterly*, 81(3): 523–50.

Black, Rachel, Marian McLaughlin, and Melanie Giles (2020), "Women's Experience of Social Media Breastfeeding Support and Its Impact on Extended Breastfeeding Success: A Social Cognitive Perspective," *British Journal of Health Psychology*, 25(3): 754–71.

Blair, Tannock (2023), "Orangutan Learns How to Nurse from Breastfeeding Zookeeper at Richmond Metro Zoo," Available online: https://www.wric.com/news/local-news/richmond/orangutan-learns-how-to-nurse-from-breastfeeding-zookeeper-at-metro-richmond-zoo/ (accessed April 2, 2023).

Blum, Linda (1999), *At the Breast: Ideologies of Breastfeeding and Motherhood in the Contemporary US*, Boston: Beacon Press.

Bourdieu, Pierre (1986), "The Forms of Capital," in J. Richardson, *Handbook of Theory and Research for the Sociology of Education*, 241–58. Westport, CT: Greenwood Press.

Boyer, Ruth (1962), "Social Structure and Socialization of the Apaches of the Mescalero Indian Reservation," PhD diss., University of California, Berkeley.

BreastfeedLA, ACLU SoCal, and California Women's Law Center (2021), "Custody and Breast/Chestfeeding Toolkit 2021," Available online: https://www.breastfeedla.org/custody-toolkit-eng-sp/ (accessed January 25, 2025).

Brewis, Alexandra, and Amber Wutich (2019), *Lazy, Crazy, and Disgusting: Stigma and the Undoing of Global Health*, Baltimore: Johns Hopkins University Press.

Budd, Kristen (2024), "Incarcerated Women and Girls," Available online: https://www.sentencingproject.org/fact-sheet/incarcerated-women-and-girls/#footnote-ref-1 (accessed December 9, 2024).

Cairns, Kathleen (2018), "JURY DUTY: Baltimore Mom Mad about Breastfeeding Accommodations," Available online: https://foxbaltimore.com/news/local/jury-duty-baltimore-mom-mad-about-breastfeeding-accommodations (accessed November 15, 2024).

Calhoun, Kendra (2016), "'What, a Black Man Can't Have a TV?': Vine Racial Comedy as a Sociopolitical Discourse Genre," M.A. thesis, Department of Linguistics, University of California, Santa Barbara. Available online: https://escholarship.org/uc/item/9wj3w192 (accessed March 3, 2025).

Calhoun, Kendra (2019), "Vine Racial Comedy as Anti-Hegemonic Humor: Linguistic Performance and Generic Innovation," *Journal of Linguistic Anthropology*, 29(1): 27–49.

Campbell, Gabriela (2022), "Language and Culture with Dr. Kendra Calhoun," That Anthro Podcast. Available online: https://creators.spotify.com/pod/profile/gabby-campbell1/episodes/Language-and-Culture-with-Dr--Kendra-Calhoun-e1bor8g (accessed April 21, 2025).

Cappellini, Benedetta, Vicki Harman, Alessandra Marilli, and Elizabeth Parsons (2019), "Intensive Mothering in Hard Times: Foucauldian Ethical Self-formation and Cruel Optimism," *Journal of Consumer Culture*, 19(4): 469–92.

Carmichael, Harris, Cindy Matsen, Phoebe Freer, Wendy Kohlmann, Matthew Stein, Saundra S. Buys, and Sarah Colonna (2017), "Breast Cancer Screening of Pregnant and Breastfeeding Women with BRCA Mutations," *Breast Cancer Research and Treatment*, 162: 225–30.

Carnino, Jonathan M., Anika S. Walia, Frances Rodriguez Lara, Amos M. Mwaura, and Jessica R. Levi (2023), "The Effect of Frenectomy for Tongue-tie, Lip-tie, or Cheek-tie on Breastfeeding Outcomes: A Systematic Review of Articles Over Time and Suggestions for Management," *International Journal of Pediatric Otorhinolaryngology*, 171: 111638. https://doi.org/10.1016/j.ijporl.2023.11163.

Carroll, Aaron (2020), "The Trouble with Growth Charts," *The New York Times*, April 17. Available online: https://www.nytimes.com/2020/04/17/parenting/growth-chart-accuracy.html (accessed July 25, 2024).

Carter, Pamela (1995). *Feminism, Breasts, and Breastfeeding*. New York: St. Martin's Press.

CDC (2022), "Breastfeeding Report Card: US 2022," Available online: https://www.cdc.gov/breastfeeding/data/reportcard.htm (accessed October 18, 2023).

CDC (2024), "CDC Museum Covid-19 Timeline," Available, online: https://www.cdc.gov/museum/timeline/covid19.html#Early-2021 (accessed March 13, 2025).

Center for Leadership Education in Maternal & Child Public Health, University of Minnesota–Twin Cities, School of Public Health (2023). *Breastfeeding and Lactation Support for Incarcerated People in the U.S.: A State Policy Brief from the National University-Based Collaborative on Justice-Involved Women and Children (JIWC)*.

Available online: https://mch.umn.edu/wp-content/uploads/2023/04/JIWC-Policy-Brief-Breastfeeding-and-Lactation-.pdf (accessed April 10, 2025).

Chandler, Mielle (2007), "Emancipated Subjectivities and the Subjugation of Mothering Practices," in Andrea O'Reilly (ed.), *Maternal Theory: Essential Readings*, 529–41, Toronto: Demeter Press.

Charnov, Eric L., and David Berrigan (1993), "Why Do Female Primates Have Such Long Lifespans and So Few Babies? Or Life in the Slow Lane," *Evolutionary Anthropology: Issues, News, and Reviews*, 1(6): 191–4.

Chary, Anita, Shom Desgupta, Sara Messmer, and Peter Rohloff (2011), "'But One Gets Tired': Breastfeeding Subjugation and Empowerment in Rural Guatemala," in Michelle Walks and Naomi McPherson (eds), *An Anthropology of Mothering*, 172–82, Bradford, ON: Demeter Press.

Chiao, Christine, Elizabeth Kaye, Thayer Scott, Catherine Hayes, and Raul I. Garcia (2021), "Breastfeeding and early childhood caries: findings from the National Health and Nutrition Examination Survey, 2011 to 2018," *Pediatric Dentistry*, 43(4): 276–81.

Claytor, Michael-Anthony (2021), "Closeted Tiktok: Liminality, Internalized Stigma, and Heterotopia in the Rite of 'Coming Out,'" Honor thesis, Department of Anthropology, Georgia State University, Atlanta, Georgia, Available online: https://hdl.handle.net/20.500.14694/501 (accessed June 12, 2025).

Clements, Dennis (2013), "Newborn Jaundice," *Duke Health*. Available online: https://www.dukehealth.org/blog/newborn-jaundice (accessed September 1, 2024).

Clements, Zakary A., Brittany N. Derr, and Sharon S. Rostosky (2022), "Male Privilege Doesn't Lift the Social Status of all Men in the Same Way: Transmasculine Individuals' Lived Experiences of Male Privilege in the United States," *Psychology of Men & Masculinities*, 23(1): 123–32.

Coleman, Barbara (2021), "Maidenform: Images of the American Woman in the 1950s," in Carol Siegel and Ann Kibbey (eds), *Genders 21: Forming and Reforming Identity*, 3–29, New York and London: New York University Press.

Copelton, Denise A, Rebecca McGee, Andrew Coco, Isis Shanbaky, and Timothy Riley (2010), "The Ideological Work of Infant Feeding," in Rhonda Shaw and Allison Bartlett (eds), *Giving Breast Milk: Body Ethics and Contemporary Breastfeeding Practice*, 24–38. Bradford, Ontario, Canada: Demeter Press.

Corley, Cheryl (2018), "Programs Help Incarcerated Moms Bond with Their Babies In Prison," *National Public Radio*. Available online: https://www.npr.org/2018/12/06/663516573/programs-help-incarcerated-moms-bond-with-their-babies-in-prison (accessed June 21, 2023).

Crittenden, Ashley N., John Sorrentino, Sheniz A. Moonie, Mika Peterson, Audax Mabulla, and Peter S. Ungar (2017), "Oral Health in Transition: The Hadza foragers of Tanzania," *PLOS One*, 12(3): e0172197.

Czosnykowska-Łukacka, Matylda, Barbara Królak-Olejnik, and Magdalena Orczyk-Pawiłowicz (2018), "Breast Milk Macronutrient Components in Prolonged Lactation," *Nutrients*, 10(12): 1893. https://doi.org/10.3390/nu10121893.

Dakshit, Anushka (2024), "Reproductive Justice Organizers in the South are Finding New Ways to Help Incarcerated Mothers," https://wagingnonviolence.org/2024/12/reproductive-justice-organizers-find-new-ways-to-help-incarcerated-mothers/ (accessed January 31, 2025).

Davis, Dána-Ain (2019), "Obstetric Racism: The Racial Politics of Pregnancy, Labor, and Birthing," *Medical Anthropology*, 38(7): 560–73.

Dettwyler, Katherine A. (1995), "A Time to Wean: The Hominid Blueprint for the Natural Age of Weaning in Modern Human Populations," in Patricia Stuart-Macadam and Katherine A. Dettwyler (eds.), *Breastfeeding: Biocultural Perspectives*, 39–73, New York: Aldine de Gruyter.

Dettwyler, Katherine A. (2004), "When to Wean: Biological Versus Cultural Perspectives," *Clinical Obstetrics and Gynecology*, 47(3): 712–23.

Dettwyler, Katherine (2009). A Worldwide Average for Weaning? Available online: https://kathydettwyler.weebly.com/a-worldwide-average-age-of-weaning----or-that-pesky-42-years-figure.html (accessed December 1, 2022).

Dettwyler, Katherine (2015), "Court Letter—Extended Breastfeeding," Available online: https://kathydettwyler.weebly.com/2015-court-letter.html (accessed January 20, 2025).

DeVane-Johnson, Stephanie, Cheryl Woods Giscombe, Ronald Williams II, Cathie Fogel, and Suzanne Thoyre (2018), "A Qualitative Study of Social, Cultural, and Historical Influences on African American Women's Infant-feeding Practices," *The Journal of Perinatal Education*, 27(2): 71–85.

Dewey, Kathryn G., Dorothy A. Finley, and Bo Lönnerdal (1984), "Breast Milk Volume and Composition during Late Lactation (7–20 months)," *Journal of Pediatric Gastroenterology and Nutrition*, 3(5): 713–20.

DeYoung, Sarah E., and Michaela Mangum (2021), "Pregnancy, Birthing, and Postpartum Experiences during COVID-19 in the US," *Frontiers in Sociology*, 6: 611212.

Douglas, Mary (1966), *Purity and Danger: An Analysis of Concepts of Purity and Taboo*, New York: Routledge.

Dowling, Sally, and David Pontin (2017), "Using Liminality to Understand Mothers' Experiences of Long-term Breastfeeding: 'Betwixt and Between', and 'Matter Out of Place'," *Health*, 21(1): 57–75.

Eidelman, Arthur I. (2021), "Breastfeeding While in Jail," *Breastfeeding Medicine*, 16(9): 663.

Emmott, Emily H., and Ruth Mace (2015), "Practical Support from Fathers and Grandmothers is associated with Lower Levels of Breastfeeding in the UK Millennium Cohort Study," *PLoS One*, 10(7): e0133547.

Evans, Brandice (2017), "Psychosocial Stress, Race, and Social Support among Breastfeeding Mothers in the American South," MA thesis, Department of Anthropology, Georgia State University, Atlanta, Georgia. Available online: https://hdl.handle.net/20.500.14694/538 (accessed July 25, 2025).

Evans, Marissa (2021), "Breastfeeding and Vaxxed: Parents Delay Weaning Children to Pass on COVID-19 Antibodies," *The L.A. Times*, 2 November. Available online: https://www.latimes.com/california/story/2021-11-02/lactating-parents-are-delaying-weaning-young-children-to-pass-on-covid-19-antibodies (accessed March 19, 2025).

Faircloth, Charlotte (2013), *Militant Lactivism: Attachment Parenting and Intensive Motherhood in the UK and France*, New York: Berghahn Books.

Feldman-Winter, Lori (2024), "Breastfeeding: AAP Policy Explained," Available online: https://www.healthychildren.org/English/ages-stages/baby/breastfeeding/Pages/Where-We-Stand-Breastfeeding.aspx (accessed July 24, 2024).

Feldman-Winter, Lori, Trina Van, Daphna Varadi, Amanda C. Adams, Bahar Kural, and Elien C. J. Rouw (2022), "Academy of Breastfeeding Medicine Position Statement: Breastfeeding as a Basic Human Right," *Breastfeeding Medicine*, 17(8): 633–4.

Fitzwater Gonzales, Laura (2018), "Framing Breastfeeding as 'Natural' and the Implication for Mothers' Identities," in Ann Marie A. Short, Abigail L. Palko, and Dionne Irving (eds), *Breastfeeding and Culture: Discourses and Representation*, 209–22, Bradford, ON: Demeter Press.

Foucault, Michel (1984), "The Means of Correct Training," excerpt from *Discipline and Punish*, in Paul Rabinow (ed.), *The Foucault Reader*, 188–205. New York: Pantheon Books.

Fouts, Hillary N. (2008), "Father Involvement with Young Children among the Aka and Bofi Foragers," *Cross-Cultural Research*, 42(3): 290–312.

Fouts, Hillary N., Barry S. Hewlett, and Michael E. Lamb (2001), "Weaning and the Nature of Early Childhood Interactions among Bofi Foragers in Central Africa," *Human Nature*, 12: 27–46.

Fouts, Hillary N., Barry S. Hewlett, and Michael E. Lamb (2005), "Parent-Offspring Weaning Conflicts among the Bofi Farmers and Foragers of Central Africa," *Current Anthropology*, 46(1): 29–50.

Freeman, Andrea (2020), *Skimmed: Breastfeeding, Race, and Injustice*, Stanford, CA: Stanford University Press.

Garðarsdóttir, Ólöf (2002), "Saving the Child: Regional, Cultural and Social Aspects of the Infant Mortality Decline in Iceland, 1770–1920," Report No. 19, *The Demoographic Data Base*, Umeå University, Umeå, Sweden.

Gary, Anna J., Erin E. Birmingham, and Laurie B. Jones (2017), "Improving Breastfeeding Medicine in Undergraduate Medical Education: A Student Survey and Extensive Curriculum Review with Suggestions for Improvement," *Education for Health*, 30(2): 163–8.

Gaynes, Atwood, and Robbie Davis-Floyd (2004), "On Biomedicine," in Carol and Melvin Ember (eds), *The Encyclopedia of Medical Anthropology: Health and Illness in the World's Cultures*, 95–108, New York: Kluwer Academic/Plenum Publishers.

GLADLAW (2025), "I Just Happen To Be A Parent Who Is Also Transgender," *GLADLAW Answers*. Available online: https://www.glad.org/tfl/stories/just-happen-parent-also-transgender/ (accessed January 19, 2025).

Glick, Peter, and Susan T. Fiske (1996), "The Ambivalent Sexism Inventory: Differentiating between Hostile and Benevolent Sexism," *Journal of Personality and Social Psychology*, 70(3): 491–512.

Glynn, Sarah Jane (2018), "An Unequal Division of Labor: How Equitable Workplace Policies Could Benefit Working Mothers," Center for American Progress. Available online: https://www.americanprogress.org/article/unequal-division-labor/ (accessed December 20, 2024).

Goffman, Erving (1963), *Stigma: Notes on the Management of Spoiled Identity*, Englewood Cliffs, NJ: Prentice-Hall.

Goldberg, Abbie E. (2013), "'Doing' and 'Undoing' Gender: The Meaning and Division of Housework in Same-sex Couples," *Journal of Family Theory & Review*, 5(2): 85–104.

Gonzalez, Emmanuel, Nicholas J. B. Brereton, Chen Li, Lilian Lopez Leyva, Noel W. Solomons, Luis B. Agellon, Marilyn E. Scott, and Kristine G. Koski (2021), "Distinct Changes Occur in the Human Breast Milk Microbiome between Early and Established Lactation in Breastfeeding Guatemalan Mothers," *Frontiers in Microbiology*, 12: 557180.

Gopalakrishna, Kathyayini P., and Timothy W. Hand (2020), "Influence of Maternal Milk on the Neonatal Intestinal Microbiome," *Nutrients*, 12(3): 823. https://doi.org/10.3390/nu12030823.

Grall, Timothy (2016), "Custodial Mothers and Fathers and Their Child Support: 2013," *US Census Bureau*. Available online: https://www.census.gov/content/dam/Census/library/publications/2016/demo/P60-255.pdf (accessed December 14, 2024).

Gray, Kathryn J., Evan A. Bordt, Caroline Atyeo, Elizabeth Deriso, Babatunde Akinwunmi, Nicola Young, Aranxta Medina Baez, Lydia L. Shook, Dana Cvrk, Kaitlyn James, Rose M. De Guzman, Sara Brigida, Khady Diouf, Ilona Goldfarb, Lisa M. Bebell, Lael M. Yonker, Alessio Fasano, Sayed A. Rabi, Michal A. Elovitz, Galit Alter, and Andrea G. Edlow (2021), "Coronavirus Disease 2019 Vaccine Response in Pregnant and Lactating Women: A Cohort Study," *American Journal of Obstetrics and Gynecology*, 225(3): 303.e1–303.e17. https://doi.org/10.1016/j.ajog.2021.03.023.

Guy, Sarit (2022), *Mommy's Hug: Weaning from Breastfeeding Together*, Self-published: Sarit Guy.

Hallonsten, A. L., L-K. Wendt, I. Mejare, D. Birkhed, C. Håkansson, A. M. Lindvall, S. Edwardsson, and G. Koch, (1996), "Dental Caries and Prolonged Breast-feeding in

18-month-old Swedish Children," *International Journal of Paediatric Dentistry*, 5(3): 149–55.

Harley, Kim, Nannette L. Stamm, and Brenda Eskenazi (2007), "The Effect of Time in the US on the Duration of Breastfeeding in Women of Mexican Descent," *Maternal and Child Health Journal*, 11(2): 119–25.

Hastrup, Kristen (1992), "A Question of Reason: Breastfeeding Patterns in Seventeenth and Eighteenth Century Iceland," in Vanessa Maher (ed.), *The Anthropology of Breast-Feeding: Natural Law or Social Construct*, 99–108, Oxfordshire: Routledge.

Hays, Sharon (1996), *The Cultural Contradictions of Motherhood*, New Haven, CT: Yale University Press.

Hewlett, Barry S., and Steve Winn (2014), "Allomaternal Nursing in Humans," *Current Anthropology*, 55(2): 200–229.

Hewlett, Bonnie (2013), *'Listen, Here is a Story': Ethnographic Life Narratives from Aka and Ngandu Women of the Congo Basin*, New York/Oxford: Oxford University Press.

Hoffman, Kelly M., Sophie Trawalter, Jordan R. Axt, and M. Norman Oliver (2016), "Racial Bias in Pain Assessment and Treatment Recommendations, and False Beliefs about Biological Differences between Blacks and Whites," *Proceedings of the National Academy of Sciences*, 113(16): 4296–301.

Horwood, Christiane, Aditi Surie, Lyn Haskins, Silondile Luthuli, Rachael Hinton, A. Chowdhury, and Nigel Rollins (2020), "Attitudes and Perceptions about Breastfeeding among Female and Male Informal Workers in India and South Africa," *BMC Public Health*, 20: 875. https://doi.org/10.1186/s12889-020-09013-9.

Humphrey, Louise T., Isabelle De Groote, Jacob Morales, Nick Barton, Simon Collcutt, Christopher Bronk Ramsey, and Abdeljalil Bouzouggar (2014), "'Earliest Evidence for Caries and Exploitation of Starchy Plant Foods in Pleistocene Hunter-gatherers from Morocco,'" *Proceedings of the National Academy of Sciences*, 111(3): 954–9.

Hunt, Katherine M., James A. Foster, Larry J. Forney, Ursel ME Schütte, Daniel L. Beck, Zaid Abdo, Lawrence K. Fox, Janet E. Williams, Michelle K. McGuire, and Mark A. McGuire, (2011) "Characterization of the Diversity and Temporal Stability of Bacterial Communities in Human Milk," *PloS One*, 6(6): e21313.

ICE (Immigration and Customs Enforcement) (2025), "Ice Issues New Policy on Pregnant, Postpartum, Nursing Individuals," Available online: https://www.ice.gov/news/releases/ice-issues-new-policy-pregnant-postpartum-nursing-individuals (accessed July 15, 2025).

Iida, Hiroko, Peggy Auinger, Ronald J. Billings, and Michael Weitzman (2007), "Association between Infant Breastfeeding and Early Childhood Caries in the US," *Pediatrics*, 120(4): e944–52.

Illich, Ivan (2003), "Medical Nemesis," *Journal of Epidemiology and Community Health*, 57(12): 919–22. (originally published 1974, in *The Lancet*).

Irby, Les'Shon (2016), "American Father Perspectives of Breastfeeding and How it Affects Breastfeeding Rates," MA thesis, School of Public Health, Georgia State

University, Atlanta, Georgia. Available online: https://hdl.handle.net/20.500.14694/9513 (accessed September 26, 2025).

Irby, Les'Shon, Emily Graybill, and Cassandra White (2019), "How Breastfeeding Behavior is Affected by the Breastfeeding Perspectives of Fathers in Georgia (USA)," *Journal of the Georgia Public Health Association*, 7(2): 85–9.

Irving, Dionne (2018), "My Black Breast Friend: Breastfeeding and my Black Body," in Ann Marie A. Short, Abigail L. Palko, and Dionne Irving (eds), *Breastfeeding and Culture: Discourses and Representation*, 128–41, Bradford, ON: Demeter Press.

Jardine, Fiona M. (2019), "Breastfeeding without Nursing: 'If Only I'd Known More About Exclusively Pumping before Giving Birth,'" *Journal of Human Lactation*, 35(2): 272–83.

Jardine, Fiona M. (2020a), "Breastfeeding Without Nursing: The Lived Experiences of Exclusive Pumpers," PhD diss., University of Maryland, College Park.

Jardine, Fiona M. (2020b), "When Available Online Support Groups Prevail: The Information Experience of Chest/Breastfeeders Who Only Express Their Milk," *Information Research*, 25(4). https://doi.org/10.47989/irisic2013.

Johnson, Helen M., and Katrina B. Mitchell, and Academy of Breastfeeding Medicine (2020), "ABM Clinical Protocol# 34: Breast Cancer and Breastfeeding," *Breastfeeding Medicine*, 15(7): 429–34.

Jubany-Roig, Pilar, and Ester Massó Guijarro (2024), "Breastfeeding Behind Bars: Experiences of Incarcerated Mothers in the Spanish Penitentiary System," *Salud Colectiva*, 20: e4665. https://doi.org/10.18294/sc.2024.4665.

Kamnitzer, Ruth (2009), "Breastfeeding in the Land of Genghis Khan," *The Natural Child Project*. Available online: https://www.naturalchild.org/articles/guest/ruth_kamnitzer.html (accessed November 19, 2022).

Keller, Erin (2023), "'I'm a Trans Dad and Breastfeed my Baby — Haters Need to Back Off,'" *New York Post*, 23 January, 2023. Available online: https://nypost.com/2023/01/23/im-a-trans-dad-and-breastfeed-my-baby-haters-need-to-back-off/ (accessed December 1, 2023).

Kleinman Arthur (1978), "Culture, Illness and Care: Clinical Lessons from Anthropologic and Cross-Cultural Research," *Annals of Internal Medicine*, 88(2): 251–8.

Knutson, Karla (2023), "The Misogyny of Lactivism: Why Breastfeeding Is Central to the Discourse of Normative Motherhood," in Andrea O'Reilly, *Normative Motherhood: Regulations, Representations, and Reclamations*, 111–28, Bradford, ON: Demeter Press.

Komisaruk, Barry R., Eleni Frangos, Wen-Ching Liu, Kachina Allen, and Stuart Brody (2011), "Women's Clitoris, Vagina, and Cervix Mapped on the Sensory Cortex: fMRI Evidence," *Journal of Sexual Medicine*, 8(10): 2822–30.

Konner, Melvin, and Marjorie Shostak (1987), "Timing and Management of Birth among the !Kung: Biocultural Interaction in Reproductive Adaptation," *Cultural Anthropology*, 2(1): 11–28.

Kreps, Sarah E., and Douglas L. Kriner (2020), "Model Uncertainty, Political Contestation, and Public Trust in Science: Evidence from the COVID-19 Pandemic," *Science Advances*, 6(43): eabd4563. https://doi.org/10.1126/sciadv.abd4563.

Kreps, Sarah E., and Douglas L. Kriner (2020), "Model Uncertainty, Political Contestation, and Public Trust in Science: Evidence from the COVID-19 Pandemic," *Science Advances*, 6(43) a Wean: The Hominid Blueprint for the Natural Age of Weaning in Modern Human Populations," in Patricia Stuart-Macadam and Katherine A. Dettwyler (eds.), *Breastfeeding: Biocultural Perspectives*, 39–73, New York: Aldine de Gruyter.

LLL International (2024a), "Breastfeeding info/Lumps and Mammograms," *La Leche League International*. Available online: https://llli.org/breastfeeding-info/lumps-and-mammograms/ (accessed July 20, 2024).

LLL International (2024b), "Breastfeeding info/Nipple-Confusion," Available online: https://llli.org/breastfeeding-info/nipple-confusion/ (accessed December 15, 2024).

LLL USA (2015), "Breastfeeding/Chestfeeding Badges Album," Available online: https://www.facebook.com/media/set/?set=a.973304546031425&type=3 (accessed October 24, 2022).

LLL USA (2021), *Facebook post*. Available online: https://www.facebook.com/LaLecheLeagueUSA/photos/pb.100064435971969.-2207520000/4397268916968287/?type=3 (accessed September 10, 2023).

Lambda Legal (2025), FAQ About Transgender Parenting (2025), "Know Your Rights: FAQ About Transgender Parenting," Available online: https://legacy.lambdalegal.org/know-your-rights/article/trans-parenting-faq (accessed January 19, 2025).

Lauro, Helen (2003), "Counterpoint: Formula Before Surgery: Is There Evidence for a New Consensus on Pediatric NPO Guidelines?" Available online: http://www3.pedsanesthesia.org/newsletters/2003summer/counterpoint.iphtml (accessed February 18, 2024).

Lawrence, Ruth (1994), *Breastfeeding: A Guide for the Medical Profession*. Maryland Heights, Missouri: Mosby Books.

Levy, David L., and André Spicer (2013), "Contested Imaginaries and the Cultural Political Economy of Climate Change," *Organization*, 20(5): 659–78.

Li, Tengfei, Baoping Ren, Dayong Li, Pingfen Zhu, and Ming Li (2013), "Mothering Style and Infant Behavioral Development in Yunnan Snub-nosed Monkeys (*Rhinopithecus bieti*) in China," *International Journal of Primatology*, 34(4): 681–95.

MacDonald, Trevor, Joy Noel-Weiss, Diana West, Michelle Walks, MaryLynne Biener, Alanna Kibbe, and Elizabeth Myler (2016), "Transmasculine Individuals' Experiences with Lactation, Chestfeeding, and Gender Identity: A Qualitative

Study," *BMC Pregnancy and Childbirth*, 16: 106. https://doi.org/10.1186/s12884-016-0907-y.

Mahoney, S. E., S. N. Taylor, and H. P. Forman (2023), "No Such Thing as a Free Lunch: The Direct Marginal Costs of Breastfeeding," *Journal of Perinatology*, 43: 678–82.

Mandalaywala, Tara M., James P. Higham, Michael Heistermann, Karen J. Parker, and Dario Maestripieri (2014), "Physiological and Behavioural Responses to Weaning Conflict in Free-ranging Primate Infants," *Animal Behaviour*, 97: 241–7.

Margolis, Maxine (1984), *Mothers and Such: Views of Women and How They Have Changed*, Berkeley: University of California Press.

Marks, Jonathan (2003), *What it Means to be 98% Chimpanzee: Apes, People, and their Genes*. Los Angeles, CA: University of California Press.

Martin-Weber, Jessica (2023), Facebook post, public site: *The Leaky Boob*. Available online: https://www.facebook.com/TheLeakyBoob/posts/pfbid02exFNvyZ67ckT XMrUkyz2zQjC7Fc67XX62LyZCvUkP7CAMHZSogmG5YjQvRprNZr1l (accessed January 15, 2023).

Mason, Mary Ann (1994), *From Father's Property to Children's Rights: The History of Child Custody in the US*, New York: Columbia University Press.

Matee, Mecky, Martin van't Hof, Sam Maselle, Frans Mikx, and Wim van Palenstein Helderman (1994). "Nursing Caries, Linear Hypoplasia, and Nursing and Weaning Habits in Tanzanian Infants," *Community Dentistry and Oral Epidemiology*, 22(5PT1): 289–93.

Maxwell, Clare, Valerie Fleming, and Lorna Porcellato (2023), "Why Have a Bottle When You Can Have Draught? Exploring Bottle Refusal by Breastfed Babies," *Maternal & Child Nutrition*, 19(2): e13481. https://doi.org/10.1111/mcn.13481.

McCombie, Susan C. (1987), "Folk Flu and Viral Syndrome: An Epidemiological Perspective," *Social Science and Medicine*, 25(9): 987–93.

McKenna, James J., and Thomas McDade (2005), "Why Babies Should Never Sleep Alone: A Review of the Co-sleeping Controversy in Relation to SIDS, Bedsharing and Breast Feeding," *Paediatric Respiratory Reviews*, 6(2): 134–52.

Mead, Margaret (2001 (original 1928), *Coming of Age in Samoa: A Psychological Study of Primitive Youth for Western Civilisation*, Boston, MA: Mariner Books.

Meek, Joan Younger, Lawrence Noble, and Section on Breastfeeding (2022), "Policy Statement: Breastfeeding and the Use of Human Milk," *Pediatrics*, 150(1): e2022057988. https://doi.org/10.1542/peds.2022-057988.

Mehta, Arpit R., Sigamani Panneer, Suparna Ghosh-Jerath, and Elizabeth F. Racine (2017), "Factors Associated with Extended Breastfeeding in India," *Journal of Human Lactation*, 33(1): 140–8.

Michigan Breastfeeding Network (2018), "Sample Letter—Breastfeeding and Custody Consideration," Available online: https://mibreastfeeding.org/wp-content/uploads/2018/11/Sample-Letter_-Breastfeeding-and-Custody-Consideration.pdf (accessed January 25, 2025).

Molitoris, Joseph (2019), "Breast-feeding During Pregnancy and the Risk of Miscarriage," *Perspectives on Sexual and Reproductive Health*, 51(3): 153–63.

Moore, Mignon (2011), *Invisible families: Gay Identities, Relationships, and Motherhood among Black Women*, Berkeley: University of California Press, 2011.

Moscone, Sherrill R., and Mary Jane Moore (1993), "Breastfeeding During Pregnancy," *Journal of Human Lactation*, 9(2): 83–8.

Moss, Peter and Guy Roberts-Holmes (2022), "Now is the time! Confronting Neoliberalism in Early Childhood," *Contemporary Issues in Early Childhood*, 23(1): 96–9.

Motherhood Beyond Bars (2025), "A Healthy Start for Infants Born to Incarcerated Women," Available online: https://www.motherhoodbeyond.org/ (accessed June 9, 2025).

Murphy, Yolanda, and Robert F. Murphy (1974), *Women of the Forest*, New York: Columbia University.

Naminara Republic (2025), "Yu Qing Cheng's Happy Sculpture Garden," Available online: https://namisum-en.imweb.me/94#lg=w20210622331039bfa0b89&slide=0 (accessed March 11, 2025).

Nardi, Gianna Maria, Roberta Grassi, Artnora Ndokaj, Michela Antonioni, Maciej Jedlinski, Gabriele Rumi, Katarzyna Grocholewicz, "Materna, Irena Dus-Ilnicka, Felice Roberto Grassi, Livia Ottolenghi, and Marta Mazur (2021), "Maternal and Neonatal Oral Microbiome Developmental Patterns and Correlated Factors: A Systematic Review—Does the Apple Fall Close to the Tree?," *International Journal of Environmental Research and Public Health*, 18(11): 5569. https://doi.org/10.3390/ijerph18115569.

National Commission on Correctional Healthcare (2023), "Breastfeeding in Correctional Settings," Available online: https://www.ncchc.org/position-statements/breastfeeding-in-correctional-settings-2023/ (accessed January 25, 2025).

National Institute of Corrections (2025), "Residential Parenting Program," Available online: https://info.nicic.gov/justice-involved-women-programs/residential-parenting-program (accessed January 25, 2025).

NIH (National Institutes of Health) (2025), "Drugs and Lactation Database," NIH/National Library of Medicine, Available online: https://www.ncbi.nlm.nih.gov/books/NBK501922/ (accessed June 1, 2025).

Nemer, David (2022), *Technology of the Oppressed: Inequity and the Digital Mundane in Favelas of Brazil*, Boston: MIT Press.

Nicolson, Nancy A. (1991), "Maternal Behavior in Human and Nonhuman Primates," in James D. Loy and Calvin B. Peters (eds), *Understanding Behavior: What Primate Studies tell us about Human Behavior*, 17–50, New York and Oxford: Oxford University Press.

O'Reilly, Andrea (2010), "Introduction," in Andrea O'Reilly (ed.), *Twenty-first-century Motherhood: Experience, Identity, Policy, Agency*, 1–19, New York: Columbia University Press.

Parker, Richard and Peter Aggleton (2003), "HIV and AIDS-related Stigma and Discrimination: A Conceptual Framework and Implications for Action," *Social Science and Medicine*, 57: 13–24.

Patel, Jilen, Robert P. Anthonappa, and Nigel M. King (2018),"All Tied Up! Influences of Oral Frenulae on Breastfeeding and their Recommended Management Strategies," *Journal of Clinical Pediatric Dentistry*, 42(6): 407–13.

Patico, Jennifer (2020), "'Of Course We'll like it, We're Kids!': Interrogating Childhood and Parenting through Children's Food," *Families, Relationships and Societies*, 9(1): 75–90.

Patico, Jennifer (2021), *The Trouble with Snack Time: Children's Food and the Politics of Parenting*, New York: NYU Press.

Peirce, Andrea (2016), "Can I Breast-Feed During Cancer Treatment," *Memorial Sloan Kettering Cancer Center*. Available online: https://www.mskcc.org/news/can-breast-feed-during-cancer-treatment (accessed June 10, 2025).

Peres, Karen Glazer, Gustavo G. Nascimento, Marco Aurelio Peres, Murthy N. Mittinty, Flavio Fernando Demarco, Ina Silva Santos, Alicia Matijasevich, and Aluisio JD Barros (2017), "Impact of Prolonged Breastfeeding on Dental Caries: A Population-based Birth Cohort Study," Pediatrics, 140(1): https://doi.org/10.1542/peds.2016-2943.

Pickert, Kate (2012), "Are You Mom Enough? Why Attachment Parenting Drives Some Mothers to Extremes—and How Dr. Bill Sears Became Their Guru," *Time*, 32–9.

Pickett, Emma (2024), *Supporting the Transition from Breastfeeding: A Guide to Weaning for Professionals, Supporters and Parents*, London: Jessica Kingsley Publishers.

Pimple, Sarah N., Michelle G. Pedler, Biehuoy Shieh, Anjali Mandava, Emily McCourt, and J. Mark Petrash (2024), "Human Breast Milk Enhances Cellular Proliferation in Cornea Wound Healing," *Current Eye Research*, 49(11): 1138–44.

Pink, Sarah, Heather Horst, Tania Lewis, Larissa Hjorth, and John Postill (2015), *Digital Ethnography: Principles and Practice*, London, Los Angeles, New Delhi: Sage Publications.

Polomeno, Viola (1999), "An Independent Study Continuing Education Program—Sex and Breastfeeding: An Educational Perspective," *The Journal of Perinatal Education*, 8(1): 29–42.

Posey, Tanius (@transking30) (2022), TikTok video. Available online: https://www.tiktok.com/@transking30/video/7121805042285350190?_r=1&_t=ZT-8uhqPxHfTw2 (accessed December 20, 2024).

Posey, Tanius (2023), "Relocate from Florida," Available online: https://www.gofundme.com/f/relocate-from-florida (accessed January 26, 2025).

Pretzel, Jillian (2022), "Are More Moms Waiting to Wean, Thanks to Covid?," *The Washington Post*, February, 1. Available online: https://www.washingtonpost.com/parenting/2022/02/01/delay-weaning-breastfeeding-covid/ (accessed November 10, 2024).

Rapley, Gill, and Tracey Murkett (2008), *Baby-led Weaning: Helping your Baby to Love Good Food*, New York City, New York: Random House.

Reich, Jennifer A. (2020), "'We Are Fierce, Independent Thinkers and Intelligent': Social Capital and Stigma Management among Mothers who Refuse Vaccines," *Social Science & Medicine*, 257: 112015.

Reid, Yvette (author) and Camilo Zepeda (illustrator) (2021), *Booby Moon: A Weaning Book for Toddlers. Creating Magic, Wonder and Ritual for a More Joyful Experience for All*, Wellington: New Zealand ISBN Agency.

Reisman, Tamar, and Zil Goldstein (2018), "Case Report: Induced Lactation in a Transgender Woman," *Transgender Health*, 3(1): 24–6.

Reuben, Lindsey (2022), "Breastfeeding Against the Clock: Motherhood on the Tenure Track," *Journal of Mother Studies*, October 1, 2022.

Robisch, Janell (2014), *To Three and Beyond: Stories of Breastfed Children and the Mothers Who Love Them*, Amarillo, Texas: Praeclarus Press.

Rosin, Hannah (2009), "The Case Against Breastfeeding," *The Atlantic*, April issue, 64–70.

Ross, Tami (2024), "Chronic Care: Illness Narratives of Parents Caring for Teens with POTS," MA thesis, Department of Anthropology, Georgia State University, Atlanta, Georgia. Available online: https://hdl.handle.net/20.500.14694/618 (accessed July 25, 2025).

Sartorius, Norman (2002), "Iatrogenic Stigma of Mental Illness: Begins with Behaviour and Attitudes of Medical Professionals, Especially Psychiatrists," *British Medical Journal*, 324(7352): 1470–1.

Sasson, Tehila (2016), "Milking the Third World? Humanitarianism, Capitalism, and the Moral Economy of the Nestlé Boycott," *The American Historical Review*, 121(4): 1196–224.

Sawyer, Wendy, and Peter Wagner (2024), "Mass Incarceration: The Whole Pie 2024," *Prison Policy Initiative*. Available online: https://www.prisonpolicy.org/reports/pie2024.html (accessed February 10, 2025).

Schafer, Ellen J., Taylor A. Livingston, Regina M. Roig-Romero, Maret Wachira, Adetola F. Louis-Jacques, and Stephanie L. Marhefka (2021), "'Breast is Best, but…' According to Childcare Administrators, not Best for the Childcare Environment," *Breastfeeding Medicine*, 16(1): 21–8.

Schnell, Alyssa (2022), "Successful Co-lactation by a Queer Couple: A Case Study," *Journal of Human Lactation*, 38(4): 644–50.

Sebitosi-Van Jaarsveld, Sandra (2022), "Cluster Feeding in Newborns and Infants: Mothers and Health Care Worker's Knowledge and Experiences," PhD diss., Stellenbosch University, Available online: http://hdl.handle.net/10019.1/125067 (accessed January 25, 2025).

Shepard, Emily C. (2024), "Many Daycares Don't Allow Breast Milk After 1 Year of Age," *Motherly*. Available online: https://www.mother.ly/news/daycares-prohibit-breast-milk/ (accessed May 12, 2025).

Shostak, Marjorie (1981), *Nisa: The Life and Words of a !Kung Woman*, New York: Random House.

Shungin, Dmitry, Simon Haworth, Kimon Divaris, Cary S. Agler, Yoichiro Kamatani, Myoung Keun Lee, Kelsey Grinde, George Hindy, Viivi Alaraudanjoki, Paula Pesonen, Alexander Teumer, Birte Holtfreter, Saori Sakaue, Jun Hirata, Yau-Hua Yu, Daniel I. Chasman, Patrik K. E. Magnusson, Takeaki Sudo, Yukinori Okada, Uwe Völker, Thomas Kocher, Vuokko Anttonen, Marja-Liisa Laitala, Marju Orho-Melander, Tamar Sofer, John R. Shaffer, Alexandre Vieira, Mary L. Marazita, Michiaki Kubo, Yasushi Furuichi, Kari E. North, Steve Offenbacher, Erik Ingelsson, Paul W. Franks, Nicholas J. Timpson, and Ingegerd Johansson (2019), "Genome-wide Analysis of Dental Caries and Periodontitis Combining Clinical and Self-reported Data," *Nature Communications*, 10: 2733. https://doi.org/10.1038/s41467-019-10630-1.

Silva, Camilla Beatriz da, Marcelly Milhomem Mendes, Bárbara Rocha Rodrigues, Thiago Lima Pereira, Denise Bertulucci Rocha Rodrigues, Virmondes Rodrigues Junior, Virginia Paes Leme Ferriani, Vinicius Rangel Geraldo-Martins, and Ruchele Dias Nogueira (2019), "Streptococcus Mutans Detection in Saliva and Colostrum Samples," *Einstein (São Paulo)*, 17(1): eAO4515. https://doi.org/10.31744/einstein_journal/2019AO4515.

Simpson, Alicia C. (2012), "Sociocultural Barriers to Breast Feeding in African American Women with Focused Intervention to Increased Prevalence," MA thesis, Department of Anthropology, Georgia State University, Atlanta, Georgia. Available online: https://hdl.handle.net/20.500.14694/11756 (accessed July 5, 2025).

Sinnott, Anne (2010), *Breastfeeding Older Children*, London: Free Association Books.

Smith, Tanya M., Christine Austin, Katie Hinde, Erin R. Vogel, and Manish Arora (2017), "Cyclical Nursing Patterns in Wild Orangutans," *Science Advances*, 3(5): e1601517. https://doi.org/10.1126/sciadv.1601517.

Staples, James (2011), "Interrogating Leprosy 'Stigma': Why Qualitative Insights are Vital," *Leprosy Review*, 82(2): 91–7.

Stevens, Emily E., Thelma E. Patrick, and Rita Pickler (2009), "A History of Infant Feeding," *The Journal of Perinatal Education*, 18(2): 32–9.

Stordal, Britta (2023), "Breastfeeding Reduces the Risk of Breast Cancer: A Call for Action in High-income Countries with Low Rates of Breastfeeding," *Cancer Medicine*, 12(4): 4616–25.

Stuart-Macadam, Patricia (1995), "Breastfeeding in Prehistory," In *Breastfeeding: Biocultural Perspectives*, Patricia Stuart-Macadam and Katherine A. Dettwyler (eds.), pp. 75-99, New York: Aldine de Gruyter.

Sugarman, Muriel, and Kathleen A. Kendall-Tackett (1995), "Weaning Ages in a Sample of American Women who Practice Extended Breastfeeding," *Clinical Pediatrics*, 34(12): 642–7.

Sugimura, Tetsu, Tomoko Seo, Nami Terasaki, Yukiko Ozaki, Noriko Rikitake, Rumiko Okabe, and Masami Matsushita, (2021), "Efficacy and Safety of Breast Milk Eye Drops in Infants with Eye Discharge," *Acta Paediatrica*, 110(4): 1322–9.

Sussex, Jasmine (2021), "Gender 'Inclusive' Language and Breastfeeding," *World Nutrition*, 12(3): 119–22.

Swaminathan, Nikhil (2007), "Strange but True: Males can Lactate," *Scientific American*. Available online: https://www.scientificamerican.com/article/strange-but-true-males-can-lactate/ (accessed October 23, 2022).

Swenson, Haley (2024), "Our Best Efforts," *Slate*. Available online: https://slate.com/human-interest/2024/03/fair-play-household-labor-division-queerness.html (accessed January 30, 2025).

Taylor, Charles (2003), *Modern Social Imaginaries*, Durham, NC: Duke University Press.

The Father's Rights Movement (2022), "Our Impact. The Father's Rights Movement," Available online: https://tfrm.org/our-impact/ (accessed January 28, 2025).

The Fed is Best Foundation (2020), "Our Mission: Safe Breastfeeding and Bottle-feeding Support," Available online: https://fedisbest.org/ (accessed August 23, 2022).

The Heritage Foundation (2024), "Mandate for Leadership: The Conservative Promise," Available online: https://static.heritage.org/project2025/2025_MandateForLeadership_FULL.pdf (accessed June 30, 2025).

Thorley, Virginia (2019), "Is Breastfeeding "Normal"? Using the Right Language for Breastfeeding," *Midwifery*, 69: 39–44.

Thorley, Virginia (2021), "Embodied Mothering: Valuing Breastfeeding in a Neoliberal Age," *Breastfeeding Review*, 29(1): 7–13.

Thulier, Diane. B (2009), "Breastfeeding in America: A History of Influencing Factors," *Journal of Human Lactation*, 25(1): 85–94.

Tomori, Cecilia, Aunchalee E. L. Palmquist, and Sally Dowling (2016), "Contested Moral Landscapes: Negotiating Breastfeeding Stigma in Breastmilk Sharing, Nighttime Breastfeeding, and Long-term Breastfeeding in the US and the UK," *Social Science & Medicine*, 168: 178–85.

Tomori, Ceclia (2021), "New Technologies Claiming to Copy Human Milk Reuse Old Marketing Tactics to Sell Baby Formula and Undermine Breastfeeding," *The Conversation*. Available online: https://theconversation.com/new-technologies-claiming-to-copy-human-milk-reuse-old-marketing-tactics-to-sell-baby-formula-and-undermine-breastfeeding-159771 (accessed April 13, 2023).

Tornello, Samantha L. (2020), "Division of Labor among Transgender and Gender Non-binary Parents: Association with Individual, Couple, and Children's Behavioral Outcomes," *Frontiers in Psychology*, 11: 15. https://doi.org/10.3389/fpsyg.2020.00015.

Townsend, Elizabeth (2024), "Trans* in the Neoliberal University: Students' Relationship with Georgia State University and its LGBTQ+ Support Structures," M.A. thesis, Department of Anthropology, Georgia State University, Atlanta, Georgia. Available online: https://hdl.handle.net/20.500.14694/616 (accessed July 1, 2025).

Trivers, Robert L. (1974), "Parent-Offspring Conflict," *American Zoologist*, 14: 249–64.

Trongsilsat, Sanpob, Jinthana Lapirattanakul, Rudee Surarit, and Apiwan Smutkeeree (2020), "In Vitro Comparison of Biofilm Formation and Acidogenicity between Human Breast Milk and other Milk Formulas," *Pediatric Dental Journal*, 30(2): 57–63.

Ukponmwan, C. U., O. T. Okolo, D. H. Kayoma, and Juliet Ese-Onakewhor (2009), "Complications of Breast Milk Application to the Infected Eye," *Nigerian Journal of Ophthalmology*, 17(1): 32–5.

USDA (US Department of Agriculture) (2024), "Special Supplemental Nutrition Program for Women, Infants, and Children (WIC)," USDA Food and Nutrition Services. Available online: https://www.fns.usda.gov/wic (accessed August 2, 2024).

Vieira, Alexandre R., Adriana Modesto, and Mary L. Marazita (2014), "Caries: Review of Human Genetics Research." *Caries Research*, 48(5): 491–506.

Volk, Anthony A. (2009), "Human Breastfeeding is not Automatic: Why That's So and What it Means for Human Evolution," *Journal of Social, Evolutionary, and Cultural Psychology*, 3(4): 305–14.

Walker, Jane R., Eileen Baldry, and Elizabeth A. Sullivan (2021), "Residential Programmes for Mothers and Children in Prison: Key Themes and Concepts," Criminology & Criminal Justice 21(1): 21–39.

Walters, Joanna (2025), "Woman in Florida Deported to Cuba Says She Was Forced to Leave Baby Daughter," *The Guardian*. Available online: https://www.theguardian.com/us-news/2025/may/02/trump-florida-mom-cuba-deported (accessed May 10, 2025).

Wayland, Coral (2004), "Infant Agency and its Implications for Breast-feeding in Brazil," *Human Organization*, 63(3): 277–88.

WBFF/Fox 45 (2018), "Breastfeeding in Jury Duty: A Mom in Southwest Baltimore is Angry over how the Baltimore City Circuit Court System Handles Jurors who are Breast Feeding," Available online: https://www.facebook.com/watch/?ref=search&v=10155553914564607&external_log_id=0f1eeb95-591f-49ac-91b2-d8cfeaef21b9&q=jury%20duty%20breastfeeding (accessed December 10, 2024).

Weerheijm, K. L., B. F. M. Uyttendaele-Speybrouck, H. C. Euwe, and H. J. Groen (1998), "Prolonged Demand Breast-feeding and Nursing Caries," *Caries Research*, 32(1): 46–50.

White, Cassandra (2008), "Iatrogenic Stigma in Outpatient Treatment for Hansen's Disease (leprosy) in Brazil," *Health Education Research*, 23(1): 25–39.

White, Cassandra (2009), *An Uncertain Cure: Living with Leprosy in Rio de Janeiro*, New Brunswick, NJ: Rutgers University Press.

White, Cassandra (2024), "'Just for Comfort': Cultural Imaginaries about Extended Breast/Chestfeeding among Medical and Legal Authorities in the U.S.," in Heidi Altman (ed), *Agency and Bodily Autonomy in Systems of Care*, 81–91, Lexington, Kentucky: Lexington Books.

Williams, Frank L'Engle (2020), *Fathers and Their Children in the First Three Years of Life: An Anthropological Perspective*, Texas: A&M University Press.

Wilson, Kristin J. (2018), *Others' Milk: The Potential of Exceptional Breastfeeding*, New Brunswick, NJ: Rutgers University Press.

Wolf, Jacqueline H. (2003), "Low Breastfeeding Rates and Public Health in the United States," *American Journal of Public Health*, 93(12): 2000–10.

Wolf, Joan B. (2011), *Is Breast Best?: Taking on the Breastfeeding Experts and the New High Stakes of Motherhood*, New York: NYU Press.

Yans-McLaughlin, Virginia, and Robert Seidman, writers; directed by Alan Berliner (1996), *Margaret Mead: An Observer Observed*, New York: Filmakers Library.

Zaikman, Yuliana, and Amy E. Houlihan (2022), "It's Just a Breast: An Examination of the Effects of Sexualization, Sexism, and Breastfeeding Familiarity on Evaluations of Public Breastfeeding," *BMC Pregnancy and Childbirth*, 22: 122. https://doi.org/10.1186/s12884-022-04436-1.

Zhinong, Xi, producer (2015), "Mystery Monkeys of Shangri-La" (documentary film), Nature/PBS Productions.

Zöllner, Maria Stella Amorim da Costa, and Antonio Olavo Cardoso Jorge (2003), "Candida spp. Occurrence in Oral Cavities of Breastfeeding Infants and in Their Mothers' Mouths and Breasts," *Pesquisa Odontológica Brasileira*, 17: 151–5.

Index

50/50 shared parenting 106

abrupt weaning 81–2
   due to breast cancer 92
   iatrogenic harm 72
Academy of Breastfeeding Medicine (ABM) 3
advertisements, *see* marketing
Africa, popular beliefs about WHO nursing recommendations for 70, *see also* Benin; Mali; Morocco; South Africa
agency 49, 81–2, *see also* child-led weaning
   infant 45, 121
   mother 61
   parent 160–1
Aggleton, Peter 20
agricultural societies 35
Aka, alloparenting 35
algorithms, social media 6
alloparenting 35, 49
allopathic medicine 71
alternative medicine, recommendations for weaning 76
AMAB ("assigned male at birth") transgender women, chest/breastfeeding 3, *see also* transgender people
American Academy of Pediatrics (AAP) 72, 86
   co-sleeping recommendations 79–80
   growth charts 78
   recommended nursing duration 55, 96–8
American Samoa 30
Anderson, Benedict, *Imagined Communities* 15
Andrews, Therese 119
anecdotal experiences, pediatric dental issues 83

anesthesia 91
anonymity, research participant 9
anthropology 49, *see also* in-depth interviews
   author positionality on research 10–11
   critical medical 72–3
   data gathering 5
   digital ethnography 2
   ethnography 4–5
   Institutional Review Board (IRB) approval 6
   medical 71
   participant observation 2, 44, 67–8, 73, 120
antibodies, breast milk 141–2
Apache 47
Appadurai, Arjun, "scapes" 157
arousal
   nursing and 129
   in nursing children 129–30
art
   representations of nursing 145–6
   in social media posts 145–6
Ashe, Leah 74
   on biomedicine 96–7
Asiodou, Ifeyinwa 161
asking for milk 132
   code words 132
   gestures 132
   paralinguistic features 134
   Sign Language 133
   terms 134
Atlantic, The 155
attachment 48, 118
Australia 7, 112
autism 60, 63
   EN and 121
autoethnography 4–5, 74, *see also* anthropology; ethnography
   author positionality 10–11
   data management 7

baby food, weaning and   22–3, see also formula
bacteria/bacterial
   communities, breast milk   85
   oral microbiome   85–6
badges, La Leche League   147
Baldwin, Elizabeth   102
Bambara   41
Bartick, Melissa   4
   on gender-inclusive terminology   3
bedsharing, see also co-sleeping
   co-sleeping and   109
beliefs about extended nursing   48, see also imaginaries
   "common sense"   15
   explanatory models   16–19
Benin   140
Bentley, Amy   22–3
Berrigan, David   42
Bertoia, Carl   106
bias
   gender   74
   healthcare   71
   judges   109
   weight   74
bilirubin   38
biomedicine   70–1, see also physicians
   Ashe on   96–7
bioremediation   24
Bird-David, Nurit   49
birthday, as milestone   122–3
Black women   5
   physicians' stereotypes about   73–4
   wet nurses   21–2
Blum, Linda   22
bodyfeeding   3
Bofi, cultural schema   48–9
books
   children's   126
   on weaning   122
booster, Covid-19   60
Borneo   44
bottle-feeding   36–8, 119–20
   breast milk   37
bottle/s
   refusal   120
   rot   82
boundary setting   131
Bourdieu, Pierre, capital   20

Boyer, Ruth   47
branch point   39–40
Brazil   45, 73, 85, 121, 139–40
   LAN houses   159
BRCA gene   93
breast cancer   141, see also mammogram
   BRCA gene   93
   nursing and   91–4
   screening   93–4
   weaning and   92
"breast is best" campaign   26–7, 152–3
breast milk   31
   antibodies   141–2
   "asking for it"   132–4
   bacterial communities   85
   bottle-feeding   37
   cavities and   83–5
   colostrum   24, 37
   donor   37
   as home remedy   139–40
   ingestion before surgery   90–1
   "invisibility"   51–2, 77
   jewelry   148
   lactoferrin   84
   macronutrients   24
   nutritional value   23–4
   storing at daycare   135
   storing at work   138
breast pump/ing   37, 55, 120, see also lactation
   mandatory breaks for   136
   "pump and dump"   90
   in the workplace   137–8
breastfeeding, see also chest/breastfeeding; extended nursing (EN); nursing
   bottle refusal   120
   "exceptional"   69–70
   policy   135, 150, 153
   relationship   37
   stigma   22
   transition to bottles   138–9
Breastfeeding Medicine   110, 138
breasts   3
   sexuality and   129
   sexualization of   24
Brewis, Alexandra, *Lazy, Crazy, and Disgusting: Stigma and the Undoing of Global Health*   74
bullying   104

Calhoun, Kendra 159
California, "Custody and Chest/breastfeeding Toolkit" 102
Canada 75, 106
Candida 85
capital
   cultural 20, 60
   economic 20
   social 20, 60
   symbolic 20
capitalism 17
Cappellini, Benedetta 155–6
caregiving
   in foraging societies 44
   shared 35, 65
Carter, Pam 8
   Breasts and Breast-feeding 128–9
case law, *Kantaras v. Kantaras* 109
cats, weaning 144–5
"cease and desist" order, nursing 103–4
censorship 159
Centers for Disease Control (CDC), growth charts 78
Central African Republic 48
Charnov, Eric 42
chemotherapy 89–90, 92
chest/breastfeeding 3, 151, *see also* extended nursing (EN)
   by Black parents 21–2
   cluster feeding 77–8
   co-lactation 107
   gender-inclusive terminology 3–4
   incarcerated women 110–14
   and pediatric dental health 80–8
   during pregnancy 88–9
   public health campaigns 26–7
   as risk factor for miscarriage 88–9
   by transgender men 3, 110
   in the United States 26–7
childcare, lived experiences 134–9
child/children, *see also* infant
   arousal while nursing 129–30
   developmental milestones 18–19
   Guardian Ad Litem (GAL) 103–4
   independence 17
   living arrangements in carceral settings 112–13
child-led weaning 1, 39–40, 45–6, 50, 61–2, 69, 103, 104, 121, 143, 153, 156

"natural" age 31
posts 123
spousal/partner support 64–6
China 41
class-based attitudes toward EN 57–8, 136
Claytor, Michael-Anthony 127
Clements, Dennis 38
climate change, imaginaries 16
cluster feeding 77–8
code words, asking for milk 132
co-lactation 107
Coleman, Barbara 24
colostrum 24, 37, 85
comments and posts 54, 151
   on abrupt weaning 72
   on arousal during nursing 129–30
   art and photographs 145–6
   on asking for breast milk 133–4
   on child-led weaning 123
   on custody and visitation following divorce 102, 103, 108
   cyberbullying 62
   on dental caries and cavities 82–3
   on EN for neurodivergent children 121
   on gentle weaning 156
   hostile sexism 62–3
   on jury duty for nursing parents 100–1
   on lactation consulting 157–8
   on milestones 146–7
   on nursing during the Covid-19 pandemic 141–2
   on nursing positions 127
   on partner/spousal support 64
   on pediatric dental issues 80–1
   positive medical encounters 94–5
   private versus public 9
   on public nursing 127–8
   sexist 25
   sharing, hesitancy 147
   stigmatizing 15
   on stigmatizing attitudes 150
   on taking medications while nursing 90
   on transgender community 151–2
   on twiddling 131, 151
   validation of lived experience 117–18

on visitation after divorce or
    separation   102
on weaning   69
conjunctivitis, breast milk as home
    remedy   140
consent, research participant   6–7
Copelton, Denise   8
Corley, Cheryl   112
cortisol   46
co-sleeping   67, 78–80, 123
    as taboo   79–80
    visitation and custody
        arrangements   107–8
cosmopolitan medicine   71
court letter   102, 103, 170–1
Covid-19   13, 139
    antibodies   141–2
    immunity   141–3
    pandemic, perceived health benefits of
        nursing during   139–44
    quarantine   160
    "science"   97
    vaccine   60, 141–2
cow's milk   22, 69
    feeding infants   33
    intolerance   55, 56
critical medical anthropology   72–3
cultural capital   20, 60
cultural schema   50
    Bofi   48–9
custody   64, 114–15
    arrangements for same-sex or gender
        fluid marriages   106–7
    court letter   102, 103, 170–1
    court opinions   105
    "equal access"   106–7
    "equal" rights   105
    Guardian Ad Litem (GAL)   103–4
    judge and lawyer familiarity with EN
        practices   108–9
    online posts concerning   102, 103,
        108
    overnight stays   103–4
    rights of the father   105–6
    separation trauma   105
    shared   109
    stepwise adaptation   107
    trans and nonbinary parents   109–10

"Custody and Chest/breastfeeding
    Toolkit"   102
cyberbullying   62

data gathering   5
data gathering, social media   7
data management, autoethnography   7
Davis, Dána-Ain   73–4
daycare   136–7
    breastfeeding policy   135–6

on-demand nursing   47, 56, 107, 121–2
dental caries/cavities   56, 60–1, 82, see
        also pediatric dental issues
    breast milk and   83–5
    in foraging societies   84
    sugar and   83–4, 86
    treatments   87–8

in-depth interviews   33, 36, 53, 54, 56,
    59, 64, 66, 68, 76, 88, 92, 104–5,
    111, 118, 120–1, 134–5, 140–1, see
    also comments and posts
    participant demographic
        profiles   166–9
    questions   163–5
Dettwyler, Katherine   42, 43, 102
    on a weaning "average"   40–1
DeYoung   160
diagnosis
    breast cancer   92–3
    mis-   73
digital ethnography   2
    Institutional Review Board (IRB)
        approval   6
    non-digital centricness   6
    openness   6
    private messaging   6–7
    self-reflection   6
discrimination
    gender   74
    racial   73–4
diversion programs   113–14, see also
        incarceration
divorce   101, see also custody; visitation
    custody and visitation after   101–10
domestic violence   104–5
donor breast milk   37, 38

Douglas, Mary, *Purity and Danger* 21
Dowling, Sally 119, 128
Drakich, Janice 106
dry nursing 122–3
duration of nursing, *see* nursing duration

earning a living, lived experiences 134–9
economic capital 20
Eidelman, Arthur 110
"electronic village" 5
Emmot, Emily 44–5
empacho 35
employee, breast pumping breaks 136, *see also* workplace
ending EN 147–8, *see also* weaning
epidemiology 73
erotophobia 24–5
estrogen 141
ethnic identity, research participant 8
ethnography 4–5, 41, 118–19, 157–8
    nursing duration in low-income women 119
exclusive breastfeeding (EBF) 3–4
explanatory models 16–17, 54–5
    based on bias or popular beliefs 73
    on extended nursing 18–19, 23–4, 70
    physicians' 73
extended family
    immigrant, negativity toward public nursing 57–8
    in the medical field, negativity toward EN 59
    mother-in-law, negativity toward EN 53–6, 60
    stepmother, negativity toward EN 57
extended nursing (EN) 1, *see also* nursing duration
    autistic children 121
    breast cancer detection and 92–3
    "cease and desist" order 103–4
    class-based attitudes toward 57–8
    commemorating 148
    "common sense" beliefs 15
    court letter 102, 170–1
    Covid-19 and 139–44
    cultural differences 29–31
    custody and visitation during 101–10
    dental caries and 86

digital ethnography 2
ending 147–8
explanatory models 16–17, 23–4, 70
    in foraging societies 44
    as intensive mothering 118–19
    last born and only children 47
    lived experience 70
    in Mongolia 29–30
    as a "natural" practice 32–4
    normalizing 152–4
    nursing aversion and 128–9
    pediatric dental issues (*see* pediatric dental issues)
    perceived health benefits 139–44
    physician recommendations 75–6
    physicians' knowledge about 72
    positive medical encounters 94–6
    public 128 (*see also* public nursing)
    spousal/partner concerns 66
    spousal/partner support 64–6
    stepmother 56–7
    stigma 1–3, 6, 12, 15, 21, 26–8, 132–3, 149–50, 154
    support 150 (*see also* support systems)
    TikTok videos 6
    time and labor costs 25–6
    twiddling 130–1

Facebook 53, 131, *see also* online support groups; posts
    LLL USA page 147
    parenting groups 5
    private groups 151
    search features 9
    support groups 7, 9, 69
Faircloth, Charlotte, *Militant Lactivism* 118–19
family, *see also* extended family
    pressure, giving in to 68
    stigmatizing attitudes from 51–2
fasting, pre-surgery 90–1
father/s 44–5, *see also* parents/parenting
    "benevolent" sexism 63
    visitation and custody rights 105–6
"Fed is Best" campaign 152–3
femininity, breasts 24
feminism, second wave 25, 105

fertility rates, in the United States   27–8
Fiske, Susan   25
flu   143
   laypersons' understanding of   73
focus groups   22, 26
folk medicine   73
food poisoning, breast milk as remedy for   139–40
foraging societies   32
   Bofi   48
   child caregiving   44
   dental issues in   84
   !Kung San   41, 47
   nursing and weaning duration   41–2, 44
   weaning practices   47–9
formula   8, 21, 22, 26, 36
   marketing   23
   regulations   161
   shortage   143
   supplementing breast milk with   38, 55, 56
Foucault, Michel   152
Fouts, Hillary   48–50
France, intensive parenting   118–19
Freeman, Andrea, *Skimmed: Breastfeeding, Race, and Injustice*   23
friends   52–3, *see also* support systems
full-term nursing (FTN)   4

gender
   -affirming care   75
   dysphoria   131–2
   identity   151
   -inclusive terminology   3–4
genetic/s   84
   testing   141
gentle weaning   39–40, 49, 57, 122, 123
Gerber baby food   23
gestures   132
Glick, Peter   25
global "average" for weaning   40–1
Goffman, Erving   19–20
Goldberg, Abbie   106
Gonzales, Laura Fitzwater   33
Gonzales, Mireya Tecpaxohitl   143
Good Housekeeping   23
gorillas, weaning   42

gradual weaning   121
Grotte de Pigeons   84
growth charts   78
guardian ad litem (GAL)   103–4
Guatemala   35, 44
Guijarro, Massó   113
guilt   69
   arousal and   129
Guy, Sarit   126
gymnurstics   126–7, 146

Hansen's disease/leprosy   20, 73, 97
   stigma   71
harm   72
hate speech   159
healthcare, bias   71, *see also* biomedicine; physicians
Hewlett, Barry   35
Hewlett, Bonnie   49
HIV/AIDS, stigma   20
holistic medicine
   dentistry   87
   recommendations for weaning   76
homo economicus   17
"homonormative" division of household labor   106
homonormativity   152
hormone/s   34
   supplements   3
hostile sexism   25, 62–3
Houlihan, Amy   24–5
human milk, *see* breast milk
human nature, Marks on   32
human right, nursing as a   100
hyperbilirubinemia   38

iatrogenesis/iatrogenic harm   71, *see also* breast cancer
   abrupt weaning   72
   through misdiagnosis   73
   through racial stereotyping   73–4
   transgender men   75
   in the UK   74
   weight bias   74
Iceland   33
identity, gender   151, 152, *see also* gender; transgender men
Illich, Ivan, *Medical Nemesis*   71

imaginaries   73, 149, *see also* explanatory
    models
  about climate change   16
  about nursing   62–3
  social   15–16
  on weaning   76
immigrant/s
  detention and deportation   110–11,
    114, 160–1
  Indian, attitude toward public
    nursing   57–8
immunity, Covid-19   141–3
immunoglobulins   23
incarceration
  breastfeeding support during   112
  "Mother Units"   113
  nursing parents in immigrant
    detention   110–11, 114
  residential programs   112–13
independence   17, 54, 62–3, 135
India   49, 135
inequality, structural   20
infant
  agency   45, 121
  co-sleeping   67, 79–80
  weight   78
initiation of nursing   34–5
Instagram   127, 159
intensive mothering, EN as   118–19
interviews   2, 4–8, 11, 51, 113, *see also*
    comments and posts; in-depth
    interviews
  on co-sleeping   79–80
  International Board Certified Lactation
    Consultant (IBCLC)   25
  virtual   54, 58
intimacy, partner/spousal   64
intolerance, cow's milk   55, 56
"invisibility" of breast milk   51–2, 77
Irby, Les'Shon   63–4
Irving, Dionne   5

Jaarsveled, Sebitosi-Van   77
jail, *see* incarceration
Jardine, Fiona   3, 5
jaundice   38
jewelry, breast milk   148
Jorge, Antonio Olavo Cardoso   85

Jubany-Roig, Pilar   113
judges, familiarity with EN practices
    108–9
jury duty
  accommodations for nursing
    parents   100–1
  deferral of service   99–101
  medical exemption   100–1

Kamnitzer, Ruth   29–30
Kendall-Tackett, Kathleen   123
K'exel Maya   44
  alloparenting   35
Kleinman, Arthur, "explanatory
    models"   16
Knutson, Karla, on "breast is best"
    campaign   26–7
Konner, Melvin   41, 47
Kreps, Sarah   97
Kriner, Douglas   97
!Kung San   41, 47

La Leche League (LLL)   55, 67, 88, 93
  badges   146–7
"lactating persons"   4
lactation
  co-   107
  courses   113–14
  room   137–8
  support   35, 38, 51, 55, 68, 80, 157–8
lactivism   156
lactoferrin   84
LAN houses   159
language
  acquisition, weaning and   132–4
  sexist   25, 62–3, 66
  verbal abuse   66
last born children, extended nursing   47
Lauro, Helen   90–1
Lawrence, Ruth, *Breastfeeding: A Guide for
    the Medical Profession*   40–1
lawyers, familiarity with EN
    practices   108–9
learning, maternal care skills   34–5
legal issues, *see* custody; jury duty; visitation
Levy, David, on imaginaries   16
Lino e Silva, Moisés   5–6
lived experience   36, 94, *see also* posts

anecdotes 83
comparative 83
extended nursing (EN) 70
gentle weaning 122–3
gymnurstics 126–7
health benefits of nursing 139–44
making a living/childcare 134–9
nursing duration 118–23
nursing during the Covid-19 pandemic 141–4
nursing while pregnant 123–6
public nursing 127–8
unexpected 117
validation 117–18
weaning 122, 132–4
long-term nursing 4
Los Angeles Times, The 143

macaques 46
Mace, Ruth 44–5
macronutrients, in breast milk 24
Mali 41
mammals
  cats, weaning 144–5
  weaning times 43–4
mammogram 1, 94
  nursing and 91–3
Mangum, Michaela 160
Margaret Mead: An Observer Observed 30
Margolis, Maxine, *Mothers and Such: Views of Women and How They Have Changed* 25–6
marketing
  formula 23
  PET Milk 23
Marks, Jonathan, on human nature 32
Martin-Weber, Jessica 131
Mason, Mary Ann 105
maternal care skills, learning 34–5
maternity leave 136, 139
Maxwell, Clare, "Why Have a Bottle when you can have Draught?" 120
McCombie, Susan 73
McKenna, James 79–80
Mead, Margaret 30, 49
media research 6
medications 89
medicine, *see also* pediatric dental issues

allopathic 71
bio- 70–1
Men's Rights Movement 105
Messenger 7
Meta 159, *see also* Facebook
Mexico 58
Michigan Breastfeeding Network 102
microaggression 73–4
microbiome 24, 84
  oral 86
milestones 42–3
  language acquisition 132–4
  posts on 146–7
  weaning 18–19, 122–3
"milkscapes" 157
miscarriage, breastfeeding as risk factor 88–9
misdiagnosis 73
misinformation 56
Molitoris, Joseph 89
Mongolia, extended nursing in 29–30
Montessori school, breastfeeding policy 135
Moore, Mignon, *Invisible Families: Gay Identities, Relationships, and Motherhood among Black Women* 106
Morocco 84
Moss, Peter 17
"Mother Units" 113
motherhood
  "good" 156
  studies 4
Motherhood Beyond Bars 110, 113–14, *see also* incarceration
mother/ing
  agency 61
  intensive, EN as 118–19
  -in law, negativity toward EN 53–6
"mothers" 4
Mundurucú 47
Murphy, Yolanda 47

Nakaya 49
National Commission on Correctional Healthcare 111–12
National Public Radio 112
"natural" practice, extended nursing as 32–4

Nemer, David   159
neoliberal/ism   16, 54
   workplace   17
networks   56
   social   76
New York Post, The   110
New York Times, The   78
night nursing   60–1, 108
   dental caries and   80–4
nipple/s
   shields   37, 63
   stimulation   129
   twiddling   130–1
nonbinary people
   chest/breastfeeding   3
   iatrogenic harm   75
non-digital centricness   6
nonhuman primates
   maternal care skills   34–5
   weaning practices   42, 46–7
normalizing EN   152–4
Norway   119
   parental leave policy   153
nursing, *see also* chest/breastfeeding; extended nursing (EN); maternal care skills; weaning
   allomaternal   35
   arousal and   129
   aversion   128–32
   branch point   39–40
   breast cancer and   91–4
   "cease and desist" order   103–4
   child agency   49
   cluster feeding   77–8
   on-demand   47, 56, 107, 121–2
   "dry"   122–3
   full-term   4
   gender-inclusive terminology   3
   as a human right   100
   independence and   62–3
   initiation   36
   long-term   4
   mammograms and   91–3
   night   60–1, 80, 108
   online support groups   5–6
   positions   126–8
   during pregnancy   123–5
   public   127–8, 143
   "reconnecting" through   136–7
   scheduled feeding   56
   setting boundaries   131
   supplementing with formula   38
   tandem   127
   visual representations   145–6
   while pregnant   88–9, 123–6
nursing duration   50
   AAP-recommended   55
   cultural differences   41
   and dental caries   86–7
   in foraging societies   41–2, 44
   global "average"   40–1
   lived experiences   118–23
   "normal"   43
   in orangutans   43–4
   "practical" support and   44–5
   US residency as predictor   58–9
   WHO recommendations   3, 70
nursing initiation   34–5
   complications   36–7
   lactation support   35, 38
   premature infants   37–8
nutritional value, breast milk   23–4

obesity, stigma   74
OB/GYN   93
   positive encounters   94–5
   weaning recommendations   88
observation, participant   2, 7, 44, 67, 73, 118
online communities   11, 50, 151
online spaces   2, 6–7, 18, 34, 52, 57, 62–3, 67–8, 98–9, 101, 118, 123
online support groups   5–6, 30, 45–6, 53, 60, 64, 68, 69, 76, 131, 150–1, 159, *see also* comments and posts
   private   62, 66
   verbal abuse   66
only children, extended nursing   47
open-mindedness, physician   94–5
openness   6
oral microbiome   86
orangutans
   maternal care skills   34–5
   nursing duration   43–4
O'Reilly, Andrea   4
overlaying   79
oxytocin   129

pacifier 36, 37
Pantley method 124
paralinguistic features, asking for milk 134
parental leave 153
parents/parenting 2, 30–1, 34, 40, *see also* custody; visitation
   agency 160–1
   in foraging societies 44
   "good" 156
   groups 5
   intensive mothering 118–19
Parker, Richard 20
participants, research
   consent 6–7
   interviews 2, 4–8, 11, 25 (*see also* in-depth interviews)
   nursing 8
   online observation 7 (*see also* observation, participant)
   pseudonyms 6–8
   race and ethnic identity 8
Pasteurization 22
paternalism 63
Patico, Jennifer 19
patriarchal societies, taboo 21
pediatric dental issues 80–1
   anecdotal experiences 83
   Candida and 85
   comparative experiences 83
   online support group posts on 82–3
   oral microbiome and 86
   and oral physiology 86
pediatrician
   advice on weaning 69, 80
   knowledge of breastfeeding 76–7
   positive encounters 95–6
   sleeping arrangement recommendations 79–80
perceived health benefits of nursing
   breast milk as home remedy 140
   Covid-19 immunity 141–3
PET Milk, marketing 23
Philippines 59
photos, in social media posts 145–6
physician, *see also* pediatrician
   explanatory models 73
   gender assumptions and biases 75
   gender-affirming care 75

knowledge about EN 72
medical excuse letter 100
open-mindedness 94–5
positive encounters 94–6
racial stereotyping 73–4
recommendations for weaning 75–6, 96–7
statements on "normal" nursing 70
weight bias 74
Pink, Sarah, *Digital Ethnography: Principles of Practice* 6
policy 71
   breast milk storage 135
   breastfeeding 135, 150
   breastfeeding support for incarcerated people 111–13
   employee break 136
   immigration 110–11, 114, 160–1
   maternity leave 136
   parental leave 153
   "return to work" 160
Polomeno, Viola 129
polycystic, ovarian syndrome 141
Pontin, David 119, 128
popular beliefs about extended nursing 18–19
Posey, Tanius 110, 132
positionality 10–11
positions, nursing 126–8
posts, *see* comments and posts
"practical" support 44–5
pregnancy 46–7, 75
   weaning during 88–9
   while nursing 123–6
premature infants, bottle-feeding 37–8
primates, *see* nonhuman primates
prison, *see* incarceration
privacy, TikTok 159
private messaging 6–7, 9, 54, 59–60, 91–2, 103
private online support groups 62, 66, 108
production, baby food 22–3
productivity 15, 17, 27, 54
prolactin 129
pseudonyms, research participant 6–8
psychiatry, iatrogenic stigma 71
public health, *see also* Covid-19; policy
   chest/breastfeeding campaigns 26–7

promoting EN as harm
    reduction   154–5
public nursing   143
    extended family resistance toward   57
    lived experience   127–8
    negative attitudes toward   24–5
    as taboo   58
Puerto Rico   46
"pump and dump"   90
pumping rooms   101

quarantine, Covid-19   160
questions, in-depth interview   163–5

race/racial
    identity   19
    participant   8
    stereotypes   73–4
Reddit   142
regulations, formula production   161
relationship, breastfeeding   37
"return to work" policy   160
Reuben, Lindsey, "Breastfeeding Against the Clock: Motherhood on the Tenure Track"   17
rhesus macaque   46
Richmond Zoo   34–5
rights of nursing parents
    custody and visitation   101–2, 105–6
    in immigrant detention   110–11
    jury duty and   99–102
Roberts-Holms, Guy   17
Robisch, Janell, *To Three and Beyond*   133–4
Ross, Tami   94
RSV (Respiratory Syncytial Virus)   143–4

same-sex couples, *see also* transgender people
    co-lactation   107
    custody and visitation arrangements   106–7
Sartorius, Norman   71
"scapes"   157
scheduled feeding   56
Scheider, Emily   100–1
Schnell, Alyssa   107
science   16
    on Covid-19   97
screening, breast cancer   93–4

search features, Facebook   9
second wave feminism   25, 105
self-reflection   6
self-weaning   45, 92, 120, *see also* child-led weaning
separation trauma   105, 171
sexism   25, 66
    "benevolent"   63
    hostile   25, 62–3
sexual intimacy, aversion   66–7
sexuality, breasts and   24, 129
shame   69, 129
shared caregiving   35, 65
shared custody   109
Shostak, Marjorie   41, 47
Sign Language, asking for milk   133
silver diamine fluoride   87–8
Simpson, Alicia   52
Sinnott, Anne, *Breastfeeding Older Children*   128
slavery   21
sleep/ing
    co-   67, 78–80, 107–8, 123
    Pantley method   124
snub-nose monkey, weaning   46
social capital   20, 60
social class, and attitudes toward EN   57–8, 68
social imaginaries, Taylor on   15–16, *see also* imaginaries
social media   4, *see also* posts
    algorithms   6
    censorship   159
    cyberbullying   62
    data gathering   7
    digital ethnography   2
    "electronic village"   5
    parenting groups   5
    support groups   5–6
    TikTok   6
solid foods   89, 120
    dental caries and   83–4
South Africa   58, 77
Spain, "Mother Units"   113
Spicer, André, on imaginaries   16
spouses/partners
    sexual intimacy aversion   66–7
    support for breastfeeding and weaning   63–4

support for EN   64–6
Staples, James, on stigma   20
stepmother, negativity toward EN   56–7
stereotypes, racial   73–4
stigma/stigmatizing attitudes   19, see also normalizing EN
    breastfeeding   22
    extended nursing (EN)   1–3, 6, 12, 15, 21, 26–8, 132–3, 149–50, 154
    from family   51–2
    Hansen's disease/leprosy   71
    HIV/AIDS   20
    iatrogenic   71
    obesity   74
    Staples on   20
    transgender   109, 151–2
storing breast milk at daycare   135
Streptococcus mutans   85, 86
stress   46, 47
    impact on weaning   43
    separation trauma   105
    visitation disputes and   102
structural inequality   20
Stuart-Macadam, Patricia   41
Sudden Infant Death Syndrome (SIDS)   78–9, 97
sugar
    in breast milk   83–4
    and dental caries   86
Sugarman, Muriel   123
Sumatra   44
support systems   5–6, 11, 150, see also family; friends; online support groups; posts
    extended family   53–63
    Facebook   7
    family   51–2
    friends   52–3
    networks   56
    private   62, 66
    public versus private comments   9
    spouses/partners   63–6
    in the workplace   17, 136–8
surgery
    anesthesia   90, 91
    fasting before   90–1
Swenson, Haley   106–7
symbolic capital   20

taboo   15, 21
    co-sleeping   79–80
    public nursing   58
tandem nursing   127, 145–6
Taylor, Charles, on social imaginaries   15–16
Thorley, Virginia   16–17, 32–3
ties   83–4, 87
TikTok   110, 127, 131, 132
    EN videos   6
    privacy concerns   159
Time   126
"time to stop"   1
Tomori, Ceclia   23, 79, 119
top surgery   75
Tornello, Samantha   106
Townsend, Elizabeth   152
transgender people   161
    chest/breastfeeding   3, 110
    child custody   109–10
    comments on   151
    gender dysphoria   131–2
    iatrogenic harm   75
    stigma   109, 151–2
trauma
    separation   105, 171
    weaning   47–8
treatment
    chemotherapy   89–90
    dental caries/cavities   87–8
tres leches (three milks)   35–6
twiddling   63, 130–1

UK, iatrogenesis   74
Ukponmwan, C. U.   140
United States
    alloparenting   35–6
    chest/breastfeeding   26–7
    co-sleeping study   79
    duration of residency as predictor of nursing duration   58–9
    fertility rates   27–8
    formula shortage   143
    Men's Rights Movement   105
    nursing duration in low-income women   119
US Immigration and Custom Enforcement (ICE)   111, see also immigrant/s

vaccine, Covid-19 60, 141–2
verbal abuse, online support group 66
Vine 159, *see also* social media
virtual interview 54, 58
visitation 101, 114–15
  arrangements for same-sex or gender fluid marriages 106–7
  co-lactation arrangement 107
  court letter 102–3, 170–1
  court opinions 105
  "equal access" 106–7
  judge and lawyer familiarity with EN practices 108–9
  night nursing 108
  online posts concerning 102–3, 108
  overnight stays 102
  rights of the father 105–6
  stepwise adaptation 107
visual representations of nursing 145–6

Washington Post, The 142–3
Wayland, Coral 45
weaning 120, 143, *see also* nursing duration
  abrupt 72, 81–2
  books on 122
  in cats 144–5
  "cease and desist" order 103–4
  child-led (*see* child-led weaning)
  coercive 49
  commercially produced baby food impact on 22–3
  cultural imaginaries 76
  due to breast cancer 92
  due to discomfort 122, 125
  in foraging societies 47–9
  gentle 39–40, 49, 57, 122, 123
  global "average" 40–1
  gradual 121
  holistic/alternative medical recommendations 76
  and independence 62–3
  language acquisition and 132–4
  lived experiences 122, 132–4
  in mammals 43–4
  milestones 18–19, 122–3
  in nonhuman primates 42, 46–7
  OB/GYN recommendations 88
  "party" 122
  pediatrician recommendations 77, 80
  physician recommendations 75–6, 96–7
  during pregnancy 88–9, 123–6
  self- 45, 92
  snub-nose monkey 46
  stress and 43
  time pressures 17, 54
weight
  bias 74
  infant 78
wet nurse 21–2
WhatsApp 159
Williams, Frank L'Engle 35
Wilson, Kristin 3, 36
  Others' Milk: The Potential of Exceptional Breastfeeding 69–70
Winn, Steve 35
Wolf, Jacqueline 22
Wolf, Joan, *Is Breast Best?* 31
women, *see* Black women
work from home 137, 144, 160
workplace
  breast pumping breaks 136–7
  daycare 136–7
  lactation room 137–8
  neoliberal 17
  parental leave policy 153
  schedule flexibility 137, 153
  storing breast milk 138
World Health Organization (WHO) 72, 154
  extended nursing recommendations 3, 70
  growth charts 78
Wutich, Amber, *Lazy, Crazy, and Disgusting: Stigma and the Undoing of Global Health* 74

X-ray, *see* mammogram

Zaikman, Yuliana 24–5
Zöllner, Maria Stella Amorim da Costa 85